Physiology of the Kidney

Lawrence P. Sullivan, Ph.D.
Professor of Physiology

Jared J. Grantham, M.D.
Professor of Medicine;
Director, Division of Nephrology

University of Kansas
College of Health Sciences
and Hospital
Kansas City, Kansas

Second Edition

LEA & FEBIGER • *Philadelphia* • *1982*

LEA & FEBIGER
600 Washington Square
Philadelphia, PA 19106
U.S.A.

Library of Congress Cataloging in Publication Data

Sullivan, Lawrence P.
    Physiology of the kidney.

    Includes index.
    1. Kidneys. I. Grantham, Jared J., 1936-
II. Title. [DNLM: 1. Kidney—Physiology.   2. Kidney   function
    tests.   WJ 102 S949p]
QP249.S84   1982   612'.463   81-18569
ISBN 0-8121-0839-6   AACR2

PRINTED IN THE UNITED STATES OF AMERICA

Print No. 3 2 1

Physiology
of the
Kidney

"*Superficially, it might be said that the function of the kidneys is to make urine; but in a more considered view one can say that the kidneys make the stuff of philosophy itself.*"

HOMER W. SMITH

Dedicated to our teachers.

PREFACE

The success of the first edition of this text suggested that preparation of a second edition was warranted. In conversations regarding possible alterations and additions, it occurred to us that the scope of the text could be broadened and improved by merging the outlook and experience of a teacher of basic science with those of a teacher of clinical science and practice. If this merger has worked, it is because both of us are primarily renal physiologists with similar interests in research. To that common foundation we have attempted to unite the expertise each of us has acquired from our different training and experience. One of us has taught physiology to first year medical students for more than twenty years. For the last twelve of those years the other has received the same students during their clinical training, has repaired the gaps in their knowledge of physiology and has taught them and house staff how to apply that knowledge to the diagnosis and treatment of disease.

The goal of the text remains the same: to teach the principles of renal physiology to medical students and physicians. We have not attempted to review or survey research in this field; rather we have tried to present a basic statement of the current knowledge of the functions of the kidney, pointing out, where necessary, the imperfections that still exist in that body of knowledge. We hope that our joint effort has enabled this second edition to approach that goal more closely and has made it more relevant to the needs of students and practitioners of medicine.

The changes in this second edition are extensive. We have changed the order in which the various topics are covered. Eight of the thirteen chapters are totally new; only three bear a close resemblance to chapters in the first edition. Two of the chapters cover topics not previously addressed: calcium, magnesium, and phosphate transport and diuretic agents. Two thirds of the figures have been replaced and 38 new figures have been added.

We are immeasurably indebted to the medical students of the University of Kansas School of Medicine for their unwitting but valuable assistance in the preparation of this text. We also wish to acknowledge the assistance of many of our colleagues at this institution. They patiently read and commented on many sections of this text. We particularly wish to thank Drs. Larry Welling and Francis Cuppage who provided the transmission electron micrographs and Dr. Andrew Evan of the University of Indiana who supplied us with the beautiful scanning electron micrographs. We wish to thank Larry Howell and the staff of the Design and Illustration Section at this institution, who beautifully and imaginatively prepared all the new illustrations for this edition. We also wish to thank Linda Carr and Helen Knefel who patiently and accurately typed all the drafts of the manuscript and Lorraine Rome who, despite our reluctance, persuaded us to accept her corrections of punctuation and sentence structure and thereby improved the quality of the final product.

Kansas City, Kansas   Lawrence P. Sullivan

                                                       Jared J. Grantham

CONTENTS

CHAPTER 1

Basic Principles

INTRODUCTION

In the process of evolution, the first simple forms of life developed in a fluid medium or environment of a constant composition, the sea. As time progressed, organisms evolved that were able to live first in fresh water and then on dry land. These organisms were able to face a hostile and everchanging external environment because they had developed mechanisms that enabled them to bathe their cells in a constant internal environment. To state it differently, these organisms could live a life relatively free and independent of changes in their external environment because of the constancy of the composition of their internal environment, their extracellular fluids. The attainment of this physiologic freedom was possible to a great extent because of the development of the kidney, the organ primarily responsible for the maintenance of the internal environment.

The kidneys accomplish this vital task in the following way. From the large volume of plasma that the circulation brings to the kidneys daily, the glomeruli filter a fluid almost identical in composition to plasma except for protein. This fluid then flows through the approximately 2,000,000 nephrons in the kidneys. The cells lining these nephrons reabsorb from this fluid specific substances in varying quantities and return them to the blood. These cells also extract additional substances from the blood and secrete them into the urine. As the kidneys perform their task, the process of glomerular filtration and all the myriad tubular mechanisms respond to a variety of factors to return to the circulation a fluid with the composition and volume required to maintain the constancy of the internal environment. In a day's time, the kidneys process the equivalent of the extracellular fluid volume of the body some 15 times by filtering approximately 40 gallons of fluid, reabsorbing from it the necessary amount of various substances and water, and adding other substances to the urine. Less than half a gallon of fluid with a vastly different composition is finally excreted.

The process of urine formation essentially consists of the transport of water and solute particles through membranes and cell layers. This transport can occur in several ways. In the glomeruli, water and solutes flow together through a porous membrane in response to hydrostatic pressure gradients. In the tubules, water and various types of solute molecules may move across cell layers in different directions at varying rates in response to a variety of forces. Common properties of the membranes and cell layers that substances must cross and basic principles of the mechanisms by which they are transported are reviewed in the following section.

STRUCTURE OF CELL MEMBRANES

Those cell membranes that have been isolated and chemically analyzed consist mainly of protein, cholesterol, and phospholipids. The phospholipids consist of a charged phosphoric end attached to a hydrocarbon chain. The polar end is hydrophilic and the hydrocarbon chain is hydrophobic. Protein molecules are thought to be mainly globular, and may also be bimodal like the phospholipids; that is, one part of the molecule is hydrophilic and the other is hydrophobic.

The lipid molecules within the membrane are arranged in two layers, as indicated in Figure 1-1. The polar hydrophilic ends are in close contact with fluid on each side of the membranes, and the hydrophobic chains are aligned away from water within the interior of the structure. These molecules are not frozen in position; rather, they are believed to move freely in any direction within the plane of the layer. Floating in this lipid layer are globular protein molecules, which may be embedded within only one layer of the lipid molecules or may extend through both layers. The polar or hydrophilic portions of these protein molecules are thought to be in contact with the solutions on either side of the lipid bilayer; the hydrophobic portions are immersed within the lipid bilayer. This construct is considered to be a highly labile, dynamic structure. Some of the protein groups may be free to move in the plane of the membrane and some may appear or disappear with time and in response to various stimuli. Other types of protein may be attached to the membrane in a more peripheral fashion on either surface. Small microfilaments may be attached to the inner surface of the membrane, assisting in holding the membrane in the shape characteristic for the particular cell type. A surface coating of carbohydrate molecules may also be attached to proteins floating in the lipid matrix.

The protein molecules within the membrane and other, extrinsic proteins that may be attached to the surface of the membrane may serve as enzymes catalyzing reactions within and without the cell. They may also serve as receptors for specific chemicals or hormones that affect cell

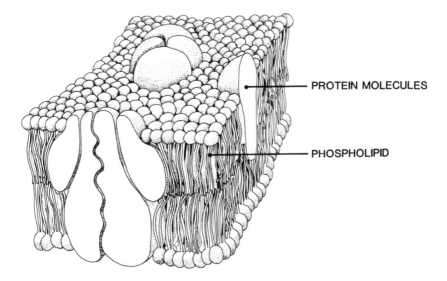

→ PROTEIN MOLECULES

→ PHOSPHOLIPID

Figure 1-1. A hypothetical view of the structure of the cell membrane. (Adapted from: Singer, S. J.: Architecture and Topography of Biologic Membranes. *In* Weissmann, G., and Clairborne, R., Eds: Cell Membranes. New York, H. P. Publishing Co., 1975; and Sweadner, K. J., and Goldin, S. M.: Active transport of sodium and potassium ions. N. Engl. J. Med. *302:*777, 1980.)

function. The nature of these proteins varies greatly among different cell types.

Molecules may enter or leave the cell through the membrane by a variety of means. Substances such as CO_2, O_2, NH_3, ethanol, and many drugs are soluble in lipid and may easily enter or leave the cell by diffusion through the lipid layer. Here, the limiting factor is not the size of the molecule but its lipid solubility. Substances that are not soluble in lipid, such as water, electrolytes, and many carbohydrates, find the lipid layer an effective barrier to diffusion. However, the protein molecules within the membrane may serve in a variety of ways to permit certain lipid-insoluble substances to cross the membrane. The structure of a protein molecule can be such that a pore or channel through the membrane is formed. The diameter of the channel may limit the size of molecules that can penetrate, but be otherwise unselective, some channels may be lined with positive or negative charges which repel ions of like charge, and others may be much more selective and accept only certain specific molecules.

The presumed diameter of these channels or pores is near the limits of resolution of the electron microscope, so anatomic evidence of their existence is not convincing. These pores may be rigid or dynamic in nature, forming and disappearing with time. Molecular size and configuration, pore diameter and ionic charge are among the factors limiting penetration by lipid-insoluble compounds through such pores or channels. These channels are thought to occupy only a small fraction of the surface area of a membrane, limiting the rate at which even the smallest lipid-insoluble substances may enter the cells by diffusion. Lipid-soluble substances, on the other hand, have available to them a large fraction of the surface area and can cross the membrane by diffusion at faster rates.

Various cells also possess special mechanisms that transport specific substances across the membrane at rates faster than can be explained by diffusion. In many instances, these mechanisms involve proteins within the membrane that serve as enzymes for chemical reactions that result in the translocation of a specific substance across the membrane.

PASSIVE DIFFUSION

The thermal energy of ions and molecules in a solution causes them to move and collide with one another in a random fashion. In a well-mixed solution, such movement does not change the concentration of the solute or solvent in any one volume unit of the solution, since molecules moving out of such a unit are replaced by molecules moving in. However, if a difference in concentration of a particular molecular species exists between two volume units or between two solutions separated by a membrane, the probability of those molecules moving from the region of high concentration to the region of low concentration exceeds the probability of the molecules moving in the opposite direction. In this situation, a net movement in one direction will take place.

In Figure 1-2 the concentration of substance X is higher in solution A than in B. The probability that molecules of X will move through pores in the membrane from A to B is higher than the probability of their moving in the opposite direction. The net flux of solute particles from A to B equals the difference between the two movements from A to B and from B to A. The magnitude of the net flux (J) of uncharged molecules per unit time is dependent on the magnitude of the concentration difference (ΔC), the permeability per unit surface area of the membrane to the solute (P), and the effective surface area (A) of the membrane available for diffusion of that particular solute. In practice, it is often difficult to determine A and it is more convenient to determine the combination of P and A, the permeability coefficient, k_p. Thus,

$$J = k_p \Delta C \tag{1-1}$$

The k_p of a membrane for a particular solute depends on the temperature; the characteristics of the membrane, such as its thickness, com-

DIFFUSION

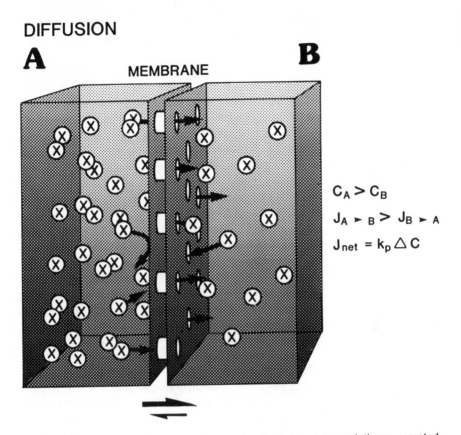

$$C_A > C_B$$

$$J_{A \rightarrow B} > J_{B \rightarrow A}$$

$$J_{net} = k_p \triangle C$$

Figure 1-2. Passive diffusion of solute molecules between two solutions separated by a permeable membrane.

position, and surface area; and the characteristics of the diffusing substance, including its size, charge, and lipid solubility.

Diffusion is the primary process by which the exchange of oxygen, carbon dioxide, nutrients, and the products of cell metabolism occurs across cell membranes and capillary membranes in all organs and tissues. It is also the major process by which drugs are absorbed from the gastrointestinal tract into the circulation and by which they reach their site of action from the circulation. Thus, molecular size, charge, and lipid solubility are among the primary determinants of the activity of many drugs. In the clinical procedure of peritoneal dialysis, diffusion is the primary mechanism for exchange of solutes across the peritoneal membrane between the circulation and the dialysate infused into the peritoneal cavity. In hemodialysis of patients with renal failure, solutes are exchanged between the patient's blood and the dialyzing fluid by diffusion across an artificial membrane. The efficacy of the artificial kidney critically depends on the selection of membrane material that will permit optimum diffusion of solutes.

MOVEMENT OF WATER THROUGH MEMBRANES

In the kidney, water moves across membranes and cell layers in response to hydrostatic pressure gradients and to osmotic pressure gradients. Under the influence of these forces, water moves through pores by a bulk or hydraulic flow process as well as by diffusion of individual molecules. The movement of fluid by hydraulic flow in response to these pressures is described in this section.

Filtration

In Figure 1-3a, a rigid membrane penetrated by pores separates two volumes of pure water. The hydrostatic pressure is higher on side A than on side B. The greater pressure on side A increases the random motion of water molecules on that side, and it may be considered that they bombard water molecules within the pore at a greater rate and with a greater force than do water molecules on side B. To state it another way, the greater activity of water molecules on side A forces water molecules within the pore into side B and a bulk flow of water takes place.

The amount of water filtered per min (J_{H_2O}) is dependent on the pressure difference across the pores (ΔP), the hydraulic permeability of the membrane, (Lp), and its surface area (A). Because of the difficulty of determining Lp and A for many biologic membranes, the product of the two is often determined. This product is called the filtration coefficient (k_f). It is an expression of the permeability of the total membrane to water and has the units of ml per min per mm Hg.
Thus,

$$J_{H_2O} = k_f \Delta P \qquad\qquad (1\text{-}2)$$

Osmosis

In Figure 1-3b two volumes of fluid under equal hydrostatic pressure are separated by a membrane permeable only to water. The fluid on side A is pure water, the fluid on side B is a solution of sucrose. Only water exists in the pores within the membrane since sucrose is too large to enter. It has been suggested that this causes a hydrostatic pressure gradient to exist along the length of the pore in the following way. Because of the size of the sucrose molecule, water molecules within the pore are subjected to collision only with water molecules on either side. A larger number of water molecules per unit volume are on side A than on side B, so the number of collisions per unit time between water

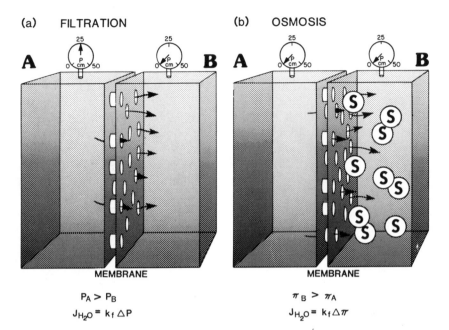

Figure 1-3. (a) Filtration of water through a permeable membrane caused by a hydrostatic pressure gradient. The pressure of each volume of water is indicated by the meter. (b) Osmotic flow of water through a semipermeable membrane caused by an osmotic concentration gradient.

molecules outside the pores and those inside will be greater on side A than on side B, and this will force water molecules within the pores into side B.

A hydrostatic pressure can be applied to side B to stop the flow of water through the pores. Again, it may be considered that this raises the rate of random movement of water molecules (the activity of water) in solution B. The increased number and force of collisions between water molecules on side B and those within the pore become equal to that on side A and thus the net flow of water through the pores becomes zero.

By definition, the osmotic pressure of the solution is that hydrostatic pressure that must be applied to it to stop the net influx of water into the solution from a volume of pure water. Remember that water flows from a region of high water concentration or activity (low solute concentration, low osmotic pressure) to a region of low water concentration or activity (high solute concentration, high osmotic pressure).

The osmotic pressure (π) of a solution is directly related to the concentration of the solute. In an ideal dilute solution

$$\pi = RTC \qquad\qquad (1\text{-}3)$$

R is the gas constant (62.3 L-mm Hg/osmole-degree), T is absolute temperature, and C is the concentration expressed in osmoles per liter. π then has the units of pressure.

The unit of osmotic mass, the osmole, is an expression of the number of solute particles in a mole of a substance. One mole of a nonionized substance such as glucose is equal to one osmole. Each molecule of a substance such as NaCl will produce two osmotic particles (Na^+ and Cl^-) when dissolved in a dilute solution. Therefore, one mole of NaCl dissolved in a large volume of water will provide two osmoles. The osmotic pressure of a solution with a concentration of one milliosmole per kilogram H_2O (mOsm/kg H_2O) at body temperature = 19.3 mm Hg or 26.2 cm H_2O (Equation 1-3).

In Figure 1-3b, the amount of water flowing from A to B per unit time, J_{H_2O}, is determined by the filtration coefficient of the membrane (k_f) and the osmotic pressure difference ($\Delta\pi$) between the two solutions.

$$J_{H_2O} = k_f \Delta\pi \qquad (1\text{-}4)$$

This equation is directly analogous to the one described earlier for filtration (Equation 1-2).

Often the movement of water across a biologic membrane other than a cell membrane results from a combination of osmotic and hydrostatic pressures. Such a situation is illustrated in Figure 1-4a. Two solutions of varying compositions are separated by a rigid, porous membrane. Solution A contains 100 mOsm/kg H_2O of urea and a hydrostatic pressure of 25 cm H_2O is exerted upon it. Solution B has the same concentration of urea, and in addition, contains 2 mOsm/kg H_2O of sucrose. A hydrostatic pressure of 50 cm H_2O is exerted upon it. The membrane has pores with a radius much larger than the radius of the urea molecules but smaller than the radius of sucrose molecules.

Solution A has a total osmotic concentration of 100 mOsm/kg H_2O, that of solution B is 102 mOsm/kg H_2O. However, the membrane will allow urea to move through it with water; thus this solute exerts no effective osmotic pressure. The only effective osmotic pressure results from the presence of sucrose. Therefore, solution A has no effective osmotic concentration ($\pi_A = 0$) and solution B has an effective osmotic concentration (π_B) of 2 mOsm/kg H_2O, or an osmotic pressure of 52.4 cm H_2O at body temperature.

Figure 1-4b illustrates the direction each pressure will tend to cause fluid to flow. The sum of the hydrostatic and osmotic pressures exerted on solution A is greater than that exerted on solution B; the net pressure difference is 27.4 cm H_2O, and that will force fluid to flow from A to B. The flow that results is a bulk flow of solution A. Since the pores are much larger than the urea molecules, urea will pass through the membrane in the stream of water. The concentration of urea in this stream

(a) OSMOSIS and FILTRATION   (b)

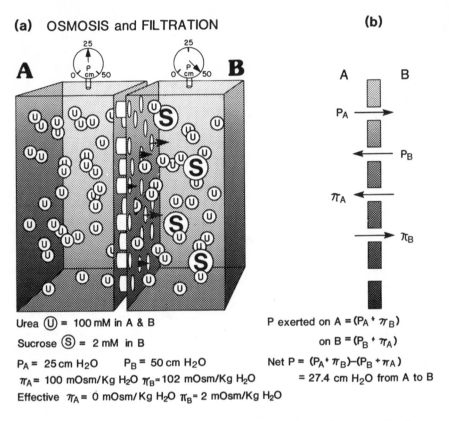

Urea U = 100 mM in A & B   P exerted on A = $(P_A + \pi_B)$

Sucrose S = 2 mM in B   on B = $(P_B + \pi_A)$

P_A = 25 cm H_2O P_B = 50 cm H_2O Net P = $(P_A + \pi_B)-(P_B + \pi_A)$

π_A = 100 mOsm/Kg H_2O π_B=102 mOsm/Kg H_2O = 27.4 cm H_2O from A to B

Effective π_A = 0 mOsm/Kg H_2O π_B= 2 mOsm/Kg H_2O

Figure 1-4.   (a) Flow of solution through a semipermeable membrane resulting from a combination of hydrostatic and osmotic pressure gradients. (b) The pressures acting to cause flow of fluid through the membrane illustrated in a.

will be the same as in solution A. Therefore, no change in the concentration of urea will take place in either solution A or B as a result of the fluid flow. Such movement of solute particles with the stream of solvent is termed solvent drag.

Reflection Coefficient

The membrane represented in Figure 1-3b was considered to be completely impermeable to the solute. In reality, few combinations of solutes and biologic membranes can be described that way. Most membranes are permeable to some extent to almost all solutes found in body fluids. Because of this, the actual or observed osmotic pressure exerted on a membrane by the presence of a substance in a solution is always somewhat less than that predicted on the basis of its concentration in the solution. The ratio of the two pressures, π_{obs}/π_{theor}, equals σ, the reflection coefficient. The upper limit of the reflection coefficient is 1.0,

and this would be the case for sucrose and the membrane in the hypothetical example illustrated in Figure 1-4. The membrane completely
"reflects" or prevents sucrose from diffusing across it. The lower limit
is zero, which would indicate that the membrane is as permeable to the
solute as it is to water. The reflection coefficient for the membrane and
urea in Figure 1-4 would approach that lower limit. The *effective* osmotic
pressures of solutions A and B exerted on that membrane can be expressed as

$$\pi_{A\,eff} = RT\sigma_u C_u$$

$$\pi_{B\,eff} = RT\sigma_u C_u + RT\sigma_s C_s$$

It is important to realize that $\pi_{A\,eff}$ and $\pi_{B\,eff}$ may be different when those
solutions are in contact with another membrane, because the reflection
coefficients of another membrane for those solutes may be different.

In practice, σ is difficult to determine, and this interrelationship between most of the solutes in body fluids and all the various membranes
has not been quantitatively measured. Qualitatively, most capillaries,
including the glomerular capillaries, are permeable to most of the electrolytes and small organic substances in plasma, and the value of σ for
these substances is small. Most capillaries are relatively impermeable to
albumin and the high molecular weight proteins. The value of σ for
these substances is substantial but less than 1.0. Only these proteins
and other foreign substances of similar size can cause an osmotic flow
of water across capillary walls.

Physiologically, the roles of filtration and osmosis and the characteristics of the membranes involved are of utmost importance in the regulation of cell volume, extracellular volume, and blood volume. Net shifts
of water between cells and extracellular fluid are thought to occur primarily by osmosis. The osmotic pressure of the extracellular fluid is
principally due to Na, Cl, and HCO_3; that of the cellular fluid is due to
K and organic anions. The reflection coefficient of the cellular membrane for these substances is difficult to determine, since specific
membrane processes, in addition to diffusion, are involved in excluding
some of these solutes from the cell and maintaining large intracellular
concentrations of others. These other membrane processes are described further on.

Both filtration and osmosis can cause net shifts of fluid between the
circulation and interstitial space across capillary walls. The pressure for
filtration is, of course, created by the heart and the direction for filtration is from the capillary into the interstitial space. Osmosis occurs
primarily in the opposite direction. As indicated earlier, the reflection
coefficient of the capillary wall for the various solutes in the extracellular
fluid is such that only substances as large as albumin can exert an

effective osmotic pressure on it. This osmotic pressure created by molecules as large as albumin is often referred to as the colloid osmotic pressure or the oncotic pressure.

In most individual capillaries, the hydrostatic pressure varies with time, and thus fluid may flow in one direction or the other across the wall as the balance between the pressures for filtration and osmosis shifts. Normally, the overall balance between the filtration or hydrostatic pressure and the colloid osmotic pressure in most capillary beds is such that little net shift of fluid occurs between plasma and interstitial fluid. Large net shifts can and do occur, however, in situations such as hemorrhage when the hydrostatic pressure falls or in diseases in which the protein concentration of the plasma is reduced.

A unique situation prevails in the capillary beds in the kidney. In the glomerular capillaries, the filtration pressure predominates, and 18 to 20% of the plasma flowing through the capillaries is filtered into the nephrons. In the peritubular capillary bed, the colloid osmotic pressure is dominant and causes a bulk flow of the fluid that has been reabsorbed from the nephrons back into the circulating plasma.

In the peritoneal dialysis procedure, glucose is often added to the dialysate because the reflection coefficient of the peritoneal membrane to glucose is sufficiently high to allow glucose to exert an effective osmotic pressure on the membrane. This counteracts the colloid osmotic pressure of the plasma and prevents the absorption of the dialysate into the circulation. In hemodialysis of patients with renal failure, it is sometimes advantageous to create a hydrostatic pressure gradient across the dialysis membrane so that filtration of plasma takes place. In this way, the patient's fluid volume can be reduced.

ELECTRICAL GRADIENTS

The electrical charge of ions in solution causes them to bind firmly a shell of water molecules. The diameter of this shell is proportional to charge density at the surface of the ion. The charge density of monovalent ions varies because the surface area of the naked ion varies. For instance, the diameter of the hydrated Na^+ ion is greater than the diameter of the hydrated Cl^- ion because the naked Na^+ ion is smaller and the charge density at the surface of the ion is greater. The hydrated radii of Cl^- and K^+ ions are approximately equal because the naked ions are about the same size.

Two important consequences arise as a result of the difference in the hydrated radii of Na^+, Cl^-, and K^+. The diffusion velocity of particles in solution is reduced by an increase in diameter, so the diffusion velocity of Na^+ is slower than the velocity of K^+ and Cl^-. Moreover, the interaction between water molecules in simple aqueous pores of membranes and those in the hydration shells permits K^+ and Cl^- to penetrate the pores more easily than Na^+.

When a crystal of NaCl is placed in a volume of water, the ions separate, acquire a hydration shell, and diffuse away from the dissolving crystal. Hydrated Cl^- ions diffuse at a faster rate than hydrated Na^+ ions because of their smaller size and tend to separate themselves from Na^+ ions. The resulting separation of charge causes the area close to the crystal to become electrically positive because the Na^+ concentration here is greater than the Cl^- concentration. Regions farther away become electrically negative because the Cl^- concentration there is greater than the Na^+ concentration.

As these ions separate, their diffusion rates are affected, because like charges or ions repel each other and unlike charges attract each other. The rate of Na^+ diffusion toward the electrically negative region is increased. Cl^- ions tend to diffuse away from the electrically positive region more slowly, and the rate of back-diffusion toward the crystal is increased. The net rate of diffusion of both ions is almost equal as a result, and there is only a microscopic separation of charge.

In a similar manner, the net diffusive flux of an ion across a membrane in response to a chemical gradient tends to separate it from ions of opposite charge, establishing an electrical potential gradient through the membrane. This electrical gradient then opposes further net diffusion of that ion.

An example of this is illustrated in Figure 1-5. A membrane permeable to Cl^- but not to Na^+ separates two solutions with unequal concentrations of NaCl. Cl^- ions diffuse in both directions across the membrane, but the flux from A to B is initially greater than the flux in the opposite direction, because of the larger concentration gradient (Fig. 1-5a). As an excess of negative ions accumulates on side B, an excess of positive charges is left on side A and an electrical potential gradient through the membrane is established.

The electrical force due to this gradient then retards the rate of diffusion of Cl^- from A to B and increases diffusion in the opposite direction (Fig. 1-5b). As time progresses, the flux of Cl^- ions down the chemical gradient from A to B raises the electrical gradient to the point where the flux of Cl^- in the opposite direction increases to the same level (Fig. 1-5c). When this point is reached, an electrochemical equilibrium is established.

It is important to realize that only a relatively small number of Cl^- ions must move from A to B to establish the electrical gradient required for equilibrium. It would be difficult to measure the actual concentration change that results in the two solutions.

What has occurred in the above example can be expressed more quantitatively. The net electrochemical energy difference ($\Delta\bar{\mu}$), representing the forces acting upon the Cl^- ion, is the algebraic sum of the chemical energy difference and the electrical energy difference across

CHLORIDE DIFFUSION POTENTIAL

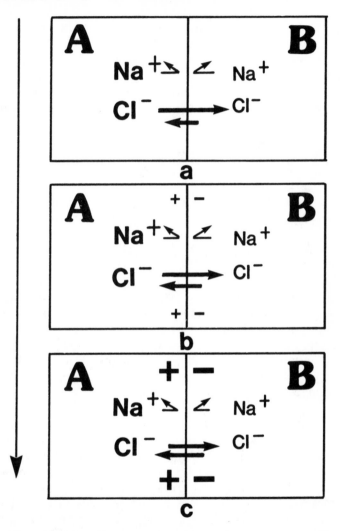

Figure 1-5. The genesis of a diffusion potential across a membrane permeable to Cl. The membrane separates two solutions of differing concentrations of NaCl. (a) Illustrates the situation immediately after the solutions are brought into contact with the membrane, (b) represents an intermediate time, and (c) illustrates the equilibrium situation. (Adapted from Vander, A. J., Sherman, J. H., and Luciano, D. S.: Human Physiology. 3rd ed. New York, McGraw-Hill, 1980.)

the membrane and can be calculated by the following equation:

$$\Delta\bar{\mu} = RT \ln \frac{C_A}{C_B} + ZFV_m \qquad (1\text{-}5)$$

R is the gas constant, T is the temperature, C_A/C_B is the ratio of the concentration of Cl^- in the two solutions, Z is the valence, F is the Faraday constant, and V_m is the electrical potential difference existing across the membrane.

When the electrical and chemical differences are equal in magnitude and opposite in direction, as in Figure 1-5c, $\Delta\bar{\mu}$ is zero and Equation 1-5 can be rearranged:

$$V_m = \frac{RT}{ZF} \ln \frac{C_A}{C_B} \qquad (1\text{-}6)$$

This is the Nernst equation. In the case of a monovalent ion and at body temperature, the Nernst equation can be simplified to

$$V_m = 61 \text{ mV} \times \log \frac{C_A}{C_B} \qquad (1\text{-}7)$$

By definition, the electrical potential difference that exists across the membrane when equilibrium for Cl^- is reached ($\Delta\bar{\mu} = 0$) is the chloride equilibrium potential, V_{Cl}.

In Figure 1-5a and b, the net amount of Cl^- moving per unit time (J_{Cl}) can be determined if the force exerted upon the Cl^- ion and the conductance of the membrane to Cl^- are known. The force is proportionate to $\Delta\bar{\mu}_{Cl}$; therefore,

$$J_{Cl} \approx g_{Cl} \Delta\bar{\mu} \qquad (1\text{-}8)$$

The conductance of the membrane to Cl^- (g_{Cl}) is a measure of the ease with which the ion can penetrate the membrane in response to the electrochemical gradient. This term is analogous to k_p, the permeability constant used in Equation 1-1 for nonionized substances, and to k_f, the filtration coefficient used in Equation 1-2. In each case, k_p, k_f, or g is a measure of the ease with which a particular substance crosses a particular membrane in response to the forces acting upon it.

Now consider a typical, nonpolar cell such as the striated muscle cell represented in Figure 1-6. The intracellular fluid contains a number of organic molecules with negative charges designated as X^-. It also has a high concentration of K^+ and low concentrations of Na^+ and Cl^-. The extracellular fluid contains high concentrations of Na^+ and Cl^- and a low concentration of K^+. The conductance to X^- is essentially nil.

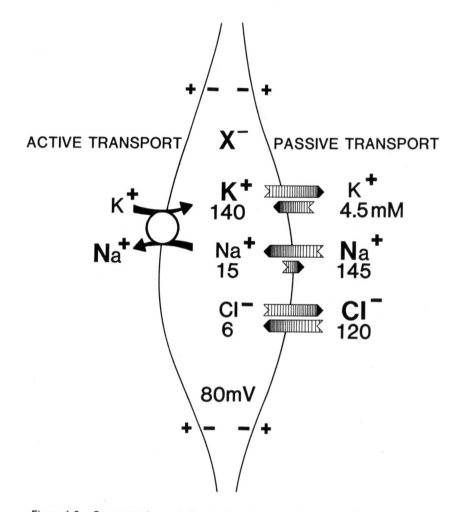

Figure 1-6. Concentration and electrical gradients and transport of ions through the membrane of a nonpolar cell such as a striated muscle cell. X^- represents impermeant anions contained within the cell.

The chemical gradient for potassium through the cell membrane causes a diffusive flux of that ion out of the cell. This flux of positive ions away from the impermeant X^- establishes an electrical gradient, which then increases the rate of K^+ diffusion into the cell and retards its outward diffusion. Measurement of the K^+ concentrations and the use of Equation 1-5 indicate that the two opposing fluxes are equal in magnitude when the membrane electrical potential difference equals 90 mV, the inside of the cell negative with respect to the outside. This is to say, $\Delta\bar{\mu}_K$ would equal zero and the V_m would equal V_K at -90 mV.

(Commonly, membrane potentials are expressed as the potential of the inside of the cell with respect to the outside.)

Measurement of the electrical potential difference with microelectrodes indicates that the actual potential difference across the membrane is less than the K^+ equilibrium potential; it averages -70 to -80 mV. Thus K^+ is not in electrochemical equilibrium. The chemical energy gradient favoring K movement out of the cell is larger than the opposing electrical energy gradient; that is, there is a net electrochemical energy difference, $(\Delta\bar{\mu}_K)$, which causes a net diffusive flux of K^+ out of the cell.

If the diffusive flux of K^+ out of the cell is greater than the diffusive flux into the cell, how is the high cellular concentration of K^+ maintained? There must be another inward flux of K^+ to balance the net outward diffusive flux. Moreover, this inward flux must occur against an electrochemical gradient, so an expenditure of energy is required to move K^+ against this gradient. For this reason and others, an active transport system is thought to reside in the membrane and to use energy supplied by the metabolism of the cell to transport K^+ inward. In this way, the net diffusive or passive flux of K^+ out of the cell is balanced by an active flux of K^+ into the cell, and the high intracellular K^+ concentration is maintained.

The chemical gradient for Na^+ favors a diffusive flux of that ion into the cell. Application of Equation 1-5 indicates that $\Delta\bar{\mu}_{Na}$ would equal zero if the membrane potential were +60 mV (V_{Na}), inside *positive* to the outside. As indicated, the actual membrane potential is -70 to -80 mV, with the inside *negative* to the outside, a difference of 100 to 110 mV. Thus, the electrical energy gradient as well as the chemical energy gradient causes Na^+ diffusion into the cell, and $\Delta\bar{\mu}_{Na}$ is relatively large. However, the amount of Na entering the cell per minute (J_{Na}) is small because g_{Na}, the conductance of the membrane to Na^+, is small. Despite the low g_{Na}, this net diffusive flux of Na^+ into the cell would, over a period of time, raise the intracellular Na^+ concentration significantly. As with K^+, it is necessary to postulate the existence of a Na^+ transport mechanism or "pump" within the membrane, which utilizes energy derived from metabolism to move Na^+ out of the cell against the electrochemical gradient.

The chemical energy gradient for Cl^- ions promotes Cl^- diffusion into the cell. However, this chemical energy gradient is approximately balanced by the opposing electrical energy gradient; $\Delta\bar{\mu}_{Cl}$ equals zero, and Cl^- is considered to be in electrochemical equilibrium.

The actual electrical potential difference across the membrane (V_m) is to a great extent the net result of the chemical energy or concentration gradients of the three principal ions that are maintained across the membrane by the "pump," and the relative conductances of the membrane to these three ions. The interrelationship among these is expressed by the following equation:

$$V_m = \frac{g_K}{\Sigma g} V_K + \frac{g_{Na}}{\Sigma g} V_{Na} + \frac{g_{Cl}}{\Sigma g} V_{Cl} \qquad (1\text{-}9)$$

in which Σg is the sum of the conductances to all ions. Depending on the circumstances and the particular type involved, other ions and charge-transporting (electrogenic) pumps may influence V_m. They have been ignored here for the sake of simplicity.

The actual V_m is far from V_{Na} (+ 60 mV) and close to V_K (-90 mV) and V_{Cl} (-80 mV) because g_K and g_{Cl} are much greater than g_{Na}. Nevertheless, the small diffusive flux of Na cations into the cell influences the V_m, keeping it somewhat smaller than V_K. The degree to which the V_m deviates from V_K is often used as a measure of the relative conductances of the membrane to K^+ and Na^+.

Renal tubular cells differ from muscle and nerve cells and differ among themselves in their permeability to Na^+, K^+, and Cl^- and in the types of transport systems they possess. As a consequence, the chemical and electrical gradients and the magnitude of the fluxes of these ions in tubular cells vary from those in muscle cells and vary from one section of the tubule to another. The transformation of a large volume of glomerular filtrate to a small volume of urine of different composition is in a large measure the result of these dissimilarities.

TYPES OF SOLUTE MOVEMENT ACROSS MEMBRANES

Solute movement across a membrane can occur in several different ways. So far, we have considered in detail the process of passive diffusion. The rate of diffusion of a solute across the membrane is determined by the lipid solubility of the solute, or its size and charge if it is not lipid-soluble, and by the electrochemical forces acting upon the solute. In this type of transport, there is no chemical interaction between the solute and components in the cell membrane, and the energy expended by the net flux of the solute is derived from whatever mechanisms established the chemical or electrical gradients.

Some solutes penetrate membranes at a rate faster than can be explained by their ability to diffuse through the membrane or by the electrochemical force acting upon them. In these circumstances, it is thought that the solute interacts or combines with some component in the cell membrane, permitting the solute to cross the membrane at a faster rate than it could otherwise.

These cell membrane components are called carriers. They are probably protein molecules or complexes of molecules imbedded in the lipid bilayer of the membrane. How the interaction between the solute and these carriers results in translocation or transport of the solute across the membrane is still very much of a mystery. One hypothesis suggests that the interaction of a solute and a membrane protein complex causes a slight change in the steric configuration of the protein such that a channel for the solute opens up. One type of carrier-mediated transport is called facilitated diffusion. The direction of transport across the membrane is determined by the electrochemical gradient for the solute, and net transport always occurs with the gradient. However, a net movement of some substances across a cell membrane has been shown to take place against an electrochemical force. Expenditure of metabolic energy is required in overcoming that force, and such processes are called active transport systems.

The two types of carrier-mediated transport, facilitated diffusion and active transport, have three distinguishing characteristics: specificity, competition, and saturation. Each transport system usually carries only a limited group of substances of the same molecular type. Within that group the different compounds compete with each other for transport by the same system. Such a transport system increases its rate of transport with a rise in the concentration of the transported substance, but only to a certain maximum. Beyond that saturation point, a further increase in concentration will not alter the transport rate.

Consider a solute that moves across a membrane by both passive diffusion and active transport. Figure 1-7 illustrates how the rate of transport by the two processes varies with the concentration of the solute. There is a simple, straightline relationship between the magnitude of the concentration and the passive flux of the substance across the membrane. However, the active transport system can increase its rate of transport only to a certain limit as the concentration of the transported substance is raised. It is thought that the number of carrier molecules limits the rate of transport. The maximum rate or velocity of active transport (V_{max}) is reached when all the available carrier molecules are combined with the transported substance. The top line represents the sum of active transport and passive diffusion. Initially, the total rate increases as the rise in solute concentration increases the rate of both processes. Above the saturation point for the active system, however, the total rate increases only as a function of the passive process.

Two useful measurements are often used to characterize carrier-mediated transport systems. One is the V_{max} and the other is the concentration of the transported substance that must be present to yield a transport rate that is one-half V_{max}. This concentration is referred to as the K_m. It can be considered to reflect the affinity of the transport system for the substance, while the V_{max} serves as an indication of the number of transporting units in a membrane.

The type of carrier mechanism involved in active transport is thought to differ from the type involved in facilitated diffusion in two ways. First, the carrier has a high affinity for the transported solute at one surface of the membrane and a low affinity at the other. Second, metabolic energy generated by the cell is utilized by the carrier in transporting solute against the electrochemical gradient.

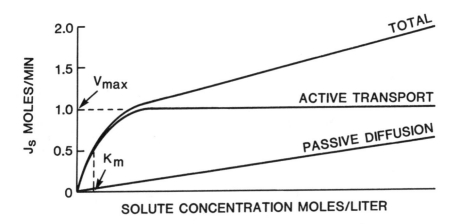

Figure 1-7. The effect of changes in solute concentration on the rate of transport of the solute by passive diffusion, by active transport, and by the sum of the two processes. V_{max} = the maximum velocity of active transport. K_m = the solute concentration required to yield an active transport rate that is one-half V_{max}.

One such active transport system that has been studied intensively is that which transports Na out of cells and K into cells. This coupled transport system, a property of the membrane of nearly all animal cells, is dependent on the presence of adenosine triphosphate (ATP) and Mg. It has now become clear that the carrier system is an integral membrane protein complex that hydrolyzes ATP as it transports Na and K. The protein complex is called Na-K activated adenosine triphosphatase (Na-K-ATPase). It is believed to be composed of two different subunits, but the molar ratio of the two units within the complex is uncertain (Fig. 1-8). The shape and molecular structure of the complex within the membrane are as yet unknown, but there is evidence that it is asymmetrically oriented in the lipid bilayer. Transport by the complex and the hydrolysis of ATP can be activated by Na and ATP only from within the cell. K acts only from the outside. Ouabain, a drug belonging to the cardiac glycoside group, is a specific inhibitor of Na-K-ATPase, and it acts only from the outside of the membrane. How combination of Na and ATP with the protein complex on the inside of the membrane and combination of K with the complex on the outside result in hydrolysis of ATP and the translocation of Na and K is still unknown. It is also not known whether Na and K are transported simultaneously or in sequence. Figure 1-8 presents a simple, hypothetical model of how this system may function.

TRANSPORT IN EPITHELIAL TISSUE

Cells in epithelial tissue such as the gastric and intestinal mucosa, gall bladder, salivary glands, and the nephron not only transport substances

Step 1

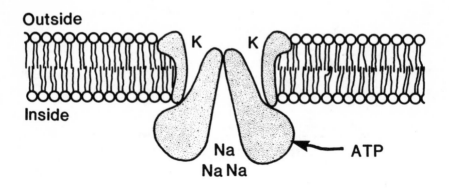

Step 2

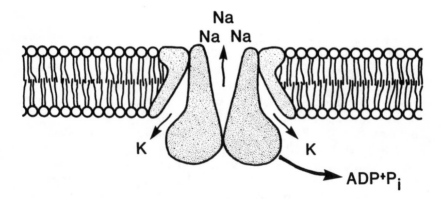

Figure 1-8.   A hypothetical representation of how Na-K-ATPase contained within the membrane may transport Na out of the cell and K in. ATP = adenosine triphosphate, ADP = adenosine diphosphate, P_i = inorganic phosphorus. (Adapted from Sweadner, K. J., and Goldin, S. M.: Active transport of sodium and potassium ions. N. Engl. J. Med. 302:777, 1980.)

between the intra- and extracellular fluids, but also transport substances from one side of the cell layer to the other. In describing this transport, it is necessary to consider the structure and organization of the cell layer as well as that of the individual cells. Figure 1-9 illustrates the basic organizational structure of many epithelial tissues. The cells are arranged in a hexagonal array in a layer that separates an external environment, such as the gastric or intestinal contents or renal tubular fluid, from the internal environment of the organism, the extracellular fluid.

Near the luminal, mucosal, or apical face of each cell, the lateral membranes of neighboring cells are fused to form a circumferential belt or layer of belts around each cell. This belt is called the zonula occludens. Its size is greatly exaggerated in the figure. The basal surface of each cell is attached to a basement membrane. The lateral surfaces of neighboring cells are separated by a fluid-filled space. This paracellular space is separated from the lumen by the zonula occludens and from the extracellular space by the basement membrane.

The microanatomy and chemical structure of the apical membrane may differ dramatically from that of the basolateral membrane. In some tissues, such as the small intestine and the proximal renal tubule, the effective surface area may be multiplied many-fold by microvillus projections into the lumen. The basolateral membrane in some tissues, such as the proximal renal tubule and thick ascending limb of the loop of Henle, may be extensively folded and interdigitated with neighboring cells so that the area of the membrane forming the wall of the paracellular space is tremendously enlarged.

The protein molecules or molecular complexes within the apical and basolateral membranes also differ both in type and quantity. For instance, receptors for the antidiuretic hormone are located in the basolateral membranes of collecting tubular cells but not in the apical membrane. Carrier complexes for organic anions and cations exist

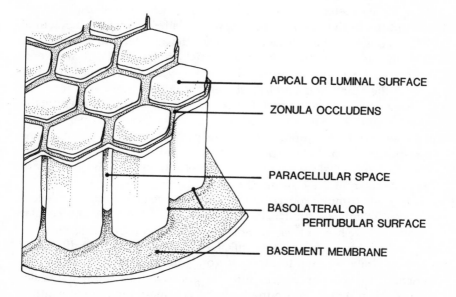

APICAL OR LUMINAL SURFACE

ZONULA OCCLUDENS

PARACELLULAR SPACE

BASOLATERAL OR
PERITUBULAR SURFACE

BASEMENT MEMBRANE

Figure 1-9. The basic structure of epithelial cell layers. The width of the zonula occludens and the paracellular space have been greatly exaggerated for purposes of emphasis.

principally in the basolateral membrane of proximal tubular cells. A carrier that transports glucose into the cell and requires the presence of Na exists in the apical membrane of proximal tubule cells. Na-K-ATPase is present in high concentration in the basolateral membrane of tubular cells, but only in small concentrations in apical membranes. It is likely that the difference in composition between the apical and basolateral membranes is the essential feature that permits these cells to transport substances across the cell layer between the external and internal environments.

The small volume of the paracellular space and the large membrane surface area in contact with it permit the cells to establish there a microenvironment whose chemical and osmotic concentration may differ substantially from the luminal fluid and the extracellular fluid. Passive transport of solutes and water may then be induced by the gradients created across the zonula occludens, the cell membranes, and the basement membrane.

The electrical properties of epithelial cell layers are highly complex. The pathway across the zonula occludens, through the paracellular space, and across the basement membrane may have a much higher conductance than the cell membranes in tissue such as the proximal tubule and the small intestine or it may have a low conductance such as in the urinary bladder and collecting tubule. Because of the differing properties of the apical and basolateral membrane, the electrical potential difference across those membranes may be substantially different. In "tight" epithelial tissues, such as the collecting tubule, these differences in the individual membrane potentials result in a large potential difference across the cell layer between the luminal and extracellular fluid, that is, the transepithelial potential difference. In "leaky" epithelial tissue, such as the proximal tubule, any large difference that may exist in the apical and basolateral membrane potentials is shunted by the high conductance paracellular pathway, so that the transepithelial potential difference may be small. In such leaky tissue, the paracellular pathway may be an important path for passive diffusion of small ions in response to small electrical or chemical gradients.

In some epithelial tissue, the transport of solutes from the lumen into the cell and from the cell into the paracellular space may cause an increase in the osmotic concentration of the paracellular fluid. The reflection coefficients of solutes in the paracellular fluid for the cellular membranes are higher than the reflection coefficients of these solutes for the basement membrane. Thus, an effective osmotic pressure difference exists to draw water into the space only from the cell and from the lumen. The flow of water into the space raises the paracellular hydrostatic pressure. Since the k_f of the basement membrane is much higher than that of the other bordering membranes, the hydrostatic pressure causes a bulk flow of water and solutes across the basement membrane into the extracellular space. Thus, the asymmetry of the structure and properties of the cell membranes, coupled with a paracellular microenvironment which is isolated from the fluid on either side of the cell layer by structures of differing properties, permit the tissue to transport net amounts of solute and water in one direction.

BIBLIOGRAPHY

General textbook references:

Davson, H. and Segal, M. B.: Introduction to Physiology. Vol 1. London, Academic Press, 1975. Chaps. 1 and 2.
DeVoe, R. D.: Principles of cell homeostasis. In Medical Physiology. 13th ed. Vol. 1. Edited by V. B. Mountcastle. St. Louis, C. V. Mosby Co., 1974.
Rapoport, S. I.: Blood-Brain Barrier in Physiology and Medicine. New York, Raven Press, 1976, Chaps 1 and 2.

Specific references for the non-specialist:

Sweadner, K. J., and Goldin, S. M.: Active transport of sodium and potassium. New Engl. J. Med., 302:777, 1980.
See also the following chapters from: Weissmann, G., and Claiborne, R., (Eds): Cell Membranes. New York, H. P. Publishing Co., 1975.
    Danielli, J. F.: The Bilayer Hypothesis of Membrane Structure.
    Singer, S. J.: Architecture and Topography of Biologic Membranes.
    Hoffman, J. F.: Ionic Transport across the Plasma Membrane.

Detailed textbook references:

Christensen, H. N.: Biological Transport. 2nd ed. Reading, Mass., W. A. Benjamin, Inc., 1975.
Dowben, R. M., Ed.: Biological Membranes. Boston, Little, Brown and Co., 1979.
Kotyk, A., and Janacek, K.: Cell Membrane Transport. New York, Plenum Press, 1970.

Detailed expositions of specific subjects:

Hebert, S. C., Schafer, J. A., and Andreoli, T. E.: Principles of Membrane Transport. In The Kidney, 2nd ed. Vol. 1. Edited by B. M. Brenner, and F. C., Rector, Jr. Philadelphia, W. B. Saunders Co., 1981.
See also the following chapters from: Andreoli, T. E., Hoffman, J. F., and Fanestil, D. D., (Eds): Physiology of Membrane Disorders. New York, Plenum Medical Book Co., 1978.
    Chapter 1. Robertson, J. D.: The Anatomy of Biological Interfaces.
    Chapter 2. Macey, R. I.: Mathematical Models of Membrane Transport Processes.
    Chapter 9. Andreoli, T. E. and Schafer, J. A.: Principles of Water and Nonelectrolyte Transport Across Membranes.
    Chapter 10. Horowicz, P., Schneider, M. F., and Begenisich, T.: Principles of Electrical Methods for Studying Membrane Movement of Ions.

Anatomy and Function of the Nephron

HISTORY OF RENAL PHYSIOLOGY

The growth of our knowledge of the anatomy and physiology of the nephron began in the seventeenth century when the first pertinent anatomic observations were made. In 1662, Lorenzo Bellini reported that the striations appearing on the cut surface of the medulla were not fibers, as was generally believed, but tubules. These were the medullary collecting ducts that today are sometimes referred to as the ducts of Bellini. Marcello Malpighi was the first to use the microscope to study renal structure. In 1666, he discovered and described the glomeruli (Malpighian corpuscles) and their connection with the renal blood vessels. Although Malpighi was the first to discover the existence of capillaries, he failed to see the glomerular capillaries. They were finally described by the Dutch worker Ruysch in 1729. Malpighi was also unable to discern the connections between the glomeruli and Bellini's ducts, but deduced that such a connection must exist and that urine formation must begin in the glomeruli.

No further notable advances in renal anatomy or physiology were made for almost two centuries, until 1842 when William Bowman published his classic observations. Utilizing a microscope with a magnifying power of x300 and a new method for injecting blood vessels, he examined the kidneys of a wide variety of species. He was able to describe precisely the glomerular capillary tuft, its spherical capsule (Bowman's capsule), the connection of the capsule with the tubule, and the single layer of cells forming the tubular wall. On the basis of these anatomic findings, Bowman developed a theory to explain the formation of urine. He considered that water escaped from the blood across the glomerular capillary wall and that this water served to flush along the tubules "urinous products" that had been secreted into the tubule by the cells lining it.

Two years later in 1844, Carl Ludwig, the great German physiologist, developed an entirely different theory. Ludwig was totally opposed to the doctrine of vitalism, which was prevalent in that era. This doctrine held that a mystical "vital force," neither physical nor chemical in nature, resides in the cells of living organisms and is ultimately responsible for all the activity of cells. Ludwig, in common with most of the astute physiologists of the nineteenth century, sought to explain all physiologic phenomena by physical and chemical principles. He believed that the idea of variable secretion of individual solutes by tubular cells was too closely allied to vitalism. Ludwig proposed an entirely mechanistic theory for urine formation. It was his view that hydrostatic pressure within the glomerular capillaries causes filtration of plasma across a highly permeable capillary wall into the capsule. The filtered fluid carries all the substances in a low concentration that are ultimately excreted in the urine in a high concentration; the filtered volume is considerably larger than the urine volume and a large fraction of the filtrate must then be reabsorbed by the tubule. Ludwig considered that filtration in the glomerular capillaries somehow concentrated the remaining blood and that this "concentrated" blood flowed on into the peritubular capillaries that surround the tubules. He proposed that the concentration of the blood created an "endosmotic" force that causes water and permeant solutes to be reabsorbed back into the blood, leaving substances such as urea to be excreted in high concentration.

Ludwig's description of this reabsorptive force was understandably rather vague. Little was known about the phenomenon of osmotic pressure at the time. The work of van't Hoff and Arrhenius was not published until the 1880s and it was not until 1896 that Starling demonstrated the osmotic effect that plasma proteins exert on water movement across capillary walls. It is also difficult to use Ludwig's theory to explain how urine may have a higher osmotic pressure than blood, but this observation was not made until 1881. Nevertheless, Ludwig was remarkably prescient. We know now that filtration is the beginning step in urine formation, that the nephron reabsorbs almost all of this fluid, that the colloid osmotic pressure of plasma entering the peritubular capillary bed is raised as a result of filtration by the glomerular capillaries, and that indeed, this pressure does play a role in the reabsorptive process, although it is by no means the only force.

There was little evidence to support any of Ludwig's thesis at the time, but soon evidence for the importance of blood pressure or blood flow in urine formation began to appear. This evidence, however, was subject to two interpretations. Rudolph Heidenhain, in studying the excretion of indigo carmine in 1874, noted that the dye could be seen in the tubular cells and tubular lumen of rabbits in which urine formation had been stopped by hemorrhage or by spinal cord transection, but could not be seen in the glomerulus. He argued that the dye is secreted from the blood into the tubule and that blood flow, not blood pressure, was important in urine formation because the tubular cells relied upon blood flow to supply the substances to be secreted. Heidenhain later calculated that in order for filtration to account for the usual amount of urea excreted daily by humans the kidneys must filter 70 L of plasma per day and reabsorb 68 L. These seemed to be impossibly large volumes. We now know, however, that the kidneys of an average man filter 180 L of fluid per day and reabsorb at least 178 L. Thus at the beginning of the twentieth century a controversy raged between proponents of the Bowman–Heidenhain theory, which to many was too closely allied with vitalism, and supporters of Ludwig's mechanistic theory.

In 1917, a monograph destined to become a landmark in the history of renal physiology was published. This monograph laid the groundwork for the first sound quantitative experiments that settled the controversy and became the foundation for modern investigation of the function of the nephron. During World War I, the eminent English physiologist Ernest Starling was editing a series of monographs on physiology and asked the Scottish pharmacologist Arthur Cushny to write one on urine formation. Cushny approached this task with vigor and a sharp razor. He stated in his preface that "No other organ of the body has suffered so much from poor work as the kidney, and in no other region of physiology does so much base coin pass as legal tender. . . . I have had to dismiss very shortly some papers which were obviously of low value." Cushny abhorred the doctrine of vitalism. He wrote: "It has the advantage that no possible conjunction can be imagined which cannot be attributed to some special activity of unspecified cells, whose activity is governed by no known laws. . . . While it offers a facile explanation of all possible observations, in reality (it) explains nothing. As a defensive position it is impregnable, but it offers no point from which advances may be made." In his preface Cushny said: "If the monograph serves as an advanced post from which others may issue against the remaining ramparts of vitalism, its purpose will be attained."

Cushny proposed a "modern view" or theory of nephron function. He accepted Ludwig's idea of filtration and then postulated that the tubules reabsorb a fluid of constant composition, a "perfected Locke's fluid." Whatever was left was then excreted. Such a process would maintain constant the composition of the extracellular fluid. Cushny absolutely refused to consider the idea that the tubules may secrete any substance whatsoever.

Cushny's monograph provided the foundation and stimulus for sound quantitative investigation of renal physiology. He ruthlessly junked much of the literature, organized the existing sound experimental evidence into a cohesive body of knowledge, and presented a largely mechanistic theory that formed a solid base for future research.

The mass of experimental evidence that ultimately validated the broad features of the Ludwig–Cushny theory was in the main provided by the monumental work of Alfred N. Richards and his co-workers at the University of Pennsylvania. With Joseph Wearn, Richards initiated and developed the technique of placing micropipets within a single glomerulus or tubular structure and withdrawing minute fluid samples which were then subjected to quantitative analysis. This technique, known today as the micropuncture technique, evolved slowly and laboriously over a period of many years, beginning in 1921. Many of the definitive papers on the composition of glomerular and tubular fluid in the amphibia did not appear until 1937. The origin of the micropuncture technique can be traced to Marshall Barber of the University of Kansas, who developed the first micromanipulators and glass micropipets for sampling small volumes of fluid. These methods, first reported in 1904, were adopted by George Kite and Robert Chambers, who in turn introduced the methodology to Richards.

Richards and Wearn first set forth to investigate the composition of the glomerular fluid, reasoning that, if it is indeed an ultrafiltrate of plasma, it should contain all the substances that exist in plasma in about the same concentration, except for protein. The development of quantitative analytic techniques for such small fluid samples (.0001 ml) was difficult. They were first able to show that the glomerular fluid in the frog kidney is essentially free of protein but contains sugar, when urine exiting from the kidney does not. Subsequently, they showed that the concentrations of glucose, phosphate, urea, uric acid, phenol red, and creatinine are substantially the same as in plasma. These observations, in conjunction with Richards' earlier work, which indicated that urine flow is indeed dependent on blood pressure but not on blood flow, and the demonstration by a co-worker, J. M. Hayman, that the hydrostatic pressure in frog glomerular capillaries exceeds the colloid osmotic pressure, proved the first tenet of the Ludwig–Cushny theory. Urine formation does indeed begin by filtration of plasma across the glomerular capillary wall into the tubule.

Subsequent work by the Philadelphia group showed that the tubules do reabsorb as both Ludwig and Cushny postulated. However, the micropuncture evidence indicated that some substances are reabsorbed in the proximal tubule but not in the distal and that the urine is made hypotonic only in the distal tubule of the amphibian nephron. Thus neither Ludwig's nor Cushny's ideas of how this reabsorption could occur were entirely correct.

What of the concept of secretion by the tubules? Cushny so abhorred the idea and tied it so tightly to the doctrine of vitalism that few wanted to consider that it existed, much less to investigate the possibility. However, Eli Marshall of Johns Hopkins was convinced that Cushny's view of secretion was unjustified, and in 1924, he and Marian Crane presented convincing evidence that phenol red is secreted by the dog kidney. Despite this, the idea of secretion was not accepted until Marshall studied the formation of urine in the marine teleost fish Lophius piscatoris. Its kidney is entirely aglomerular and made up wholly of blind tubules; substances can be added to the urine only by secretion. In later years of course, it became clear that the mammalian kidney secretes a variety of organic compounds as well as K, H, and NH_3. Thus, the 80- to 90-year long controversy over the Bowman–Heidenhain and Ludwig–Cushny theories was finally settled, and as so often happens in scientific disputes, both theories were found to contain elements of truth. Filtration and reabsorption are the predominant features of urine formation, but the tubular cells do secrete and this process is important to the kidney's role of maintaining the constancy of the composition of the internal environment.

With this conceptual framework in hand, it became possible to see a way to measure renal function quantitatively. This was a necessity, not only for the physiologist studying the mechanisms of filtration, reabsorption, and secretion, but also for the clinical scientist attempting to study the response of the kidney to disease. Indeed, much of the impetus for the development of these techniques came from clinical medicine. The concept of clearance, that is, the volume of blood cleared of a substance by the kidney per unit time, developed slowly as clinicians attempted to study the factors affecting the excretion of urea. Donald Van Slyke and his co-workers were instrumental in developing the clearance concept as it applied to urea.

Poul Rehberg in Copenhagen and Homer Smith at New York University independently recognized the value of using the clearance concept to measure the rate of glomerular filtration. What was needed was a substance that is easily filtered but not transported at all by the tubule, so that the amount entering the tubule by filtration equalled the amount excreted in the urine. Rehberg considered that creatinine met these requirements, but later work showed that creatinine is secreted to some extent. Smith examined a variety of carbohydrates, and ultimately both he and Richards independently hit upon the idea of using inulin, an inert polysaccharide with a molecular weight of about 5000. Experiments in both Smith's and Richard's laboratories showed that inulin did indeed meet all the necessary criteria.

The ability to measure the filtration rate makes it possible to measure the quantity of a substance entering the nephrons at the glomeruli; coupling this with a measurement of what leaves the collecting ducts permits a quantitative measurement of tubular activity whether it be secretion or reabsorption. Smith and his co-workers proceeded to make full use of this tool to study and measure tubular function. They found a substance, Diodrast, that was secreted from the blood so avidly that its rate of excretion could be used to determine the rate of renal blood flow.

They were also able to devise measurements of the total quantity of functional tubular tissue. This work became the foundation on which many others were to build in studying glomerular and tubular function in health and disease.

Smith exerted a tremendous influence on renal physiology not only because of his work but also through his writings and his students. Among the latter were Robert Pitts and Robert Berliner, who established productive laboratories at Cornell and at the National Institutes of Health, and James Shannon, who guided the U.S. National Institutes of Health during a remarkable period of explosive growth in biomedical research during the years following World War II.

ANATOMY OF RENAL CIRCULATION

The arterial network of the kidney is illustrated in Figure 2-1. The renal artery branches into several interlobar arteries (not shown) and thence into arcuate arteries that run along the boundary between the cortex and the medulla. The arcuate arteries send parallel branches out through the cortex towards the capsule. These are the interlobular arteries from which are derived the afferent arterioles that supply the glomeruli.

The renal circulatory system possesses the unique feature of two capillary beds arranged in series and separated only by the efferent arteriole. The first in the series, the glomerular capillaries, empties into the efferent arteriole which conveys the blood to the second capillary bed, the peritubular capillaries. Over much of the length of the glomerular capillaries, the hydrostatic pressure of the plasma is higher than the colloid osmotic pressure. Thus the balance of these two opposing pressures favors filtration. In the peritubular capillary bed, downstream from the efferent arteriole, the hydrostatic pressure is low and the opposing colloid osmotic pressure has risen as a result of filtration of protein-free fluid from the glomerular capillaries. This causes absorption of fluid from the interstitial space, fluid that had been reabsorbed from the tubules.

In the superficial cortex and mid-cortex, the peritubular capillaries form networks that surround all the cortical tubular structures. In the juxtamedullary region, the efferent arterioles branch after leaving the glomeruli. Some of these branches immediately divide into peritubular capillary networks in the outer medulla where they surround loops of Henle and collecting tubules. Others form bundles of vessels that penetrate deep into the medulla before branching (Fig. 2-1). It is important to note that in the superficial and mid-cortex blood perfusing the glomeruli comes into contact with proximal tubular tissue, but in the juxtamedullary region blood may flow from the glomeruli directly into the medulla. The usual means of measuring renal blood flow involves the use of a substance that is secreted from the blood into the tubular fluid

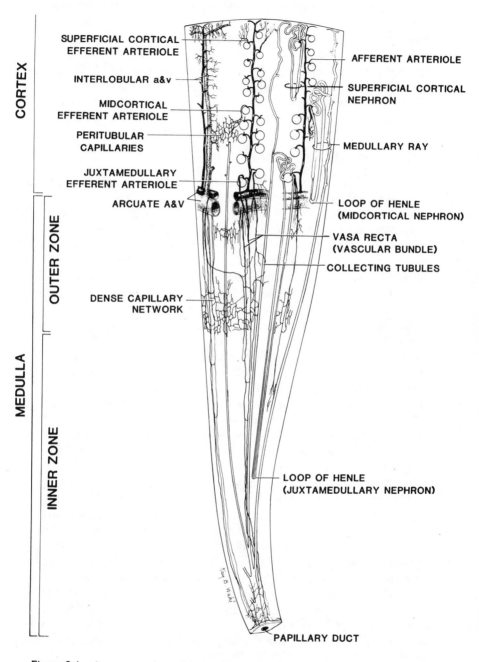

SUPERFICIAL CORTICAL
EFFERENT ARTERIOLE

AFFERENT ARTERIOLE

INTERLOBULAR a&v

SUPERFICIAL CORTICAL
NEPHRON

MIDCORTICAL
EFFERENT ARTERIOLE

PERITUBULAR
CAPILLARIES

MEDULLARY RAY

JUXTAMEDULLARY
EFFERENT ARTERIOLE

LOOP OF HENLE
(MIDCORTICAL NEPHRON)

ARCUATE A&V

VASA RECTA
(VASCULAR BUNDLE)

COLLECTING TUBULES

DENSE CAPILLARY
NETWORK

LOOP OF HENLE
(JUXTAMEDULLARY NEPHRON)

PAPILLARY DUCT

CORTEX

MEDULLA

OUTER ZONE

INNER ZONE

Figure 2-1. A cross section of the renal architecture

31

by proximal tubular cells. The assumption is made that all the blood flowing through the kidney is perfusing proximal tubular tissue. Obviously, this assumption is not entirely correct.

It is important to reiterate that the glomerular and peritubular capillary beds are arranged in series. There is no shunting of blood flow from the interlobular arteries directly into the peritubular capillary bed or into the venous drainage. Consequently, diseases that cause swelling and inflammation of the glomerular capillaries may have a profound effect on renal blood flow.

ANATOMY OF THE TUBULAR NETWORK

Figure 2-2 illustrates the major segments of the nephron. The glomerular filtrate flows from the glomerular capsule into the proximal tubule, which superficially is composed of two major sections: an initial convoluted portion, the pars convoluta, and then a straight segment, the pars recta, which descends toward the medulla. Close examination of the cell types in the proximal tubule has indicated that actually three segments exist: S_1, the initial segment of the pars convoluta, S_2, the intermediate segment, which includes the rest of the pars convoluta and the beginning of the pars recta, and S_3, the rest of the pars recta.

The tubular fluid then enters the hairpin loop of Henle, which can be divided into the thin segment and the thick segment. The loop of Henle conducts the urine flow towards or through the medulla and then directs it towards the surface of the cortex. At the end of the thick, ascending limb of the loop, the tubular fluid comes into contact through the tubular wall with the same glomerulus from which it originated and with the afferent and efferent arterioles attached to the glomerulus. The confluence of these structures forms the juxtaglomerular apparatus. This is the major site of control of the rates of renal blood flow and glomerular filtration. Specialized cells in the apparatus also secrete the enzyme renin, which is involved in the control of arterial blood pressure.

From the loop of Henle, the tubular fluid flows into the convoluted distal tubule and mixes with tubular fluid from other nephrons as several distal tubules join to form the collecting tubules. Functionally and anatomically, the distal tubule is a region of transition. The early segment is essentially an extension of the ascending limb and the later section is the beginning of the collecting tubules. The collecting tubules carry the tubular fluid straight down from the cortex through the medulla into the papilla. The urine then exits into the renal pelvis. The collecting tubule is composed of three sections that differ in structure and function: the cortical, outer medullary, and inner medullary segments.

Figure 2-2 also illustrates the differences between the cortical nephrons that originate near the surface of the kidney and the juxtamedullary nephrons that begin near the border between the cortex and medulla of

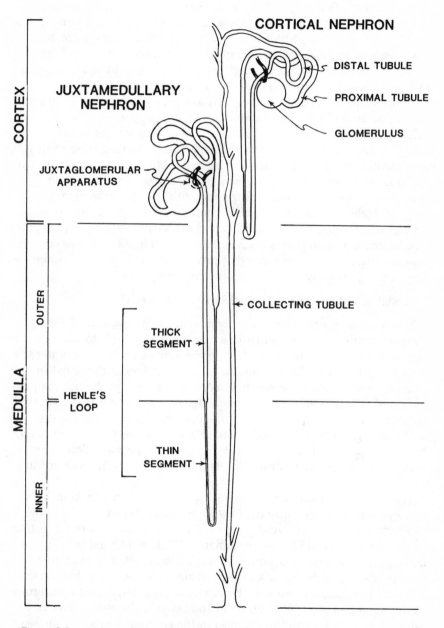

CORTICAL NEPHRON

JUXTAMEDULLARY NEPHRON

DISTAL TUBULE

PROXIMAL TUBULE

GLOMERULUS

JUXTAGLOMERULAR APPARATUS

CORTEX

MEDULLA

OUTER

INNER

HENLE'S LOOP

THICK SEGMENT →

THIN SEGMENT →

← COLLECTING TUBULE

Figure 2-2.   Anatomy of the nephrons

the kidney. The major anatomic difference is the length of the loops of Henle. The thin segment of the loop in cortical nephrons is short and the thick segment often begins before the bend in the loop. These loops do not extend into the medulla. In addition, the proximal convoluted tubules of cortical nephrons are shorter and the glomeruli are smaller than those of juxtamedullary nephrons. The relative number of the two types of nephrons varies among different species. In man, approximately 12% of the nephrons are of the juxtamedullary type.

Figure 2-1 illustrates such nephrons as they might appear in situ in a section of the kidney. The glomeruli and the proximal and distal convoluted tubules of these and all other nephrons are confined to the cortex, whereas only the loops of Henle and collecting tubules of the juxtamedullary nephrons enter the medulla. Most of the active work of the kidney is performed by the tubular structures in the cortex and this part of the kidney is profusely supplied with blood. In the medulla, the long, straight, parallel loops of Henle, coupled with a blood supply carried also in long loops, establish and maintain there a unique extracellular environment that is characterized by high salt and urea concentrations and osmotic pressures that profoundly influence the composition of the urine flowing through the collecting tubules.

GENERAL FEATURES OF GLOMERULAR FUNCTION

The process of urine formation begins at the glomerulus. In the glomerular capillaries, the hydrostatic pressure forces 18 to 20% of the plasma to filter through a complex membranous structure and enter the nephron. This ultrafiltrate contains all the substances that exist in the plasma, in the same concentration as in plasma except the plasma proteins and substances bound to the proteins. Normally, the filtrate contains only a trace of protein. Since the proteins are not filtered, the loss of the filtrate raises the protein concentration of the plasma remaining in the capillaries. The consequent increase in plasma colloid osmotic pressure opposes the hydrostatic pressure and limits the rate of filtration.

Table 2-1 lists some of the quantities involved in filtration by the kidneys of an average individual weighing 70 kg. Normally, the kidneys receive over 1700 L of blood per day. Of the plasma contained in that blood, the glomeruli filter approximately 180 L or 42.5 gal per day containing, among other substances, about 2.5 lb of salt, 0.11 lb of urea and 0.36 lb of sugar. It is the task of the tubules then, acting in response to a variety of stimuli, to excrete about half of the filtered urea and return all the sugar and over 99% of the salt and water to the circulation. At the same time, they respond to changes in the composition and volume of the extracellular fluid in such a way that the fluid returned to the circulation, the tubular reabsorbate, has the volume and composition required to maintain constant the composition and volume of the extracellular fluid, our internal environment.

TABLE 2-1   QUANTITIES INVOLVED IN URINE FORMATION IN THE HUMAN*

Fluid:
Renal Blood Flow, RBF = 1200 ml/min (20 to 25% of cardiac output)
Renal Plasma Flow, RPF = 660 ml/min
Glomerular Filtration Rate, GFR = 125 ml/min
Fraction of plasma flow filtered, GFR/RPF = 0.18-0.20

Solutes:

	Plasma Concen-tration mM	Filtered/day mmoles	g	Excreted/day mmoles	g	Percent Reabsorbed
Sodium	140	25,200	570	103	2.3	99+
Chloride	105	18,900	660	103	3.7	99+
Bicarbonate	25	4,500	275	2	0.1	99+
Potassium	4	720	30	100	4.2	86+
Glucose	5	900	160	trace		100
Urea	5	900	50	360	20.0	60
Urate	0.3	54	9	4	0.7	93
Water		180 L		1 – 1.5 L		99+

*Average values for a man weighing 70 kg.

GENERAL FEATURES OF TUBULAR FUNCTION

After plasma is filtered and the ultrafiltrate enters the nephron, a variety of forces operate to alter the concentration of substances in that fluid and the amount of each that is excreted. The reabsorption of water tends to cause the concentration of all substances in the tubular fluid to increase, and there are a few substances whose concentration changes only for this reason. They do not interact with or cross the tubular wall to a significant extent. The amount of these substances that is excreted is virtually equal to the amount that is filtered. The polysaccharide inulin is one such substance. Among others are cyanocobalamin or vitamin B_{12} and iothalamate.

Most of the naturally occurring constituents of the filtrate are reabsorbed to varying extents across the tubular wall and returned to the blood stream. This reabsorption may occur passively down an electrochemical gradient or it may be accomplished actively by specific transport processes residing in the tubular cells. The amount of each of these substances that is excreted is always less than the amount filtered. Their concentration in the final urine may be greater or smaller than their concentration in the filtrate, depending on the relative degrees to which they and water are reabsorbed.

Some substances gain entrance to the tubule not only by filtration but by secretion, that is, by crossing the tubular wall from the blood perfusing the tubules. The concentration of these substances in the urine is greater than in the glomerular filtrate and the amount excreted exceeds the amount that is filtered. Among such compounds are hippurate, penicillin, thiamine, and saccharin.

A few substances, such as potassium and uric acid, are both reabsorbed and secreted by the tubular epithelium, and their concentration in the urine and the amount excreted vary greatly. The tubular cells also can secrete into the tubular fluid the products of enzymatic reactions that take place within them. Two such substances are hydrogen ions and ammonia.

The movement of substances in either direction across the tubular epithelium can occur by passive diffusion or by active transport. The net flux of a substance in one direction is often the result of a combination of these processes. This is the situation with gradient-limited or "pump-leak" systems. For instance, the active transport of Na out of the nephron tends to reduce the concentration in the tubular fluid. A chemical gradient then exists for passive diffusion into the tubule. The *net* reabsorptive rate is determined by the difference in the rates of the active and passive processes. The rate of passive diffusion or "back-leak" into the tubule depends on the conductance of the tubular wall for Na (g_{Na}) as well as on the electrochemical gradient (Equation 1-8). In any one segment of the nephron where g_{Na} is constant, the major limitation on the *net* rate of transport is the electrochemical gradient driving the "back-leak" rather than the capacity of the pump. This is true also for the transport of K, Cl, H, and certain other inorganic ions. Both the conductance and the electrochemical gradient for each of these ions vary greatly along the length of the nephron and vary in any one segment in different circumstances. Other substances with a larger molecular radius and a low degree of lipid solubility, such as glucose, phosphate, para-aminohippurate, and penicillin usually do not diffuse across the tubular wall in significant amounts. Thus the *net* transport of these substances is limited to only a slight extent by "back-leaks" down concentration gradients. These transport systems can be shown to be limited to a much greater extent by the capacity of the active transport pathway.

All of the tubular transport systems are interdependent to a varying extent. One important transport mechanism influences the rate of transport of many solutes because it exerts a significant influence on their electrochemical gradients. This is active Na reabsorption, which utilizes a large fraction of the total energy supply to the kidney. First, this transport process permits the maintenance of electrical gradients across the luminal and peritubular cell membranes and the electrical gradient across the entire tubular epithelium. These gradients in turn affect the rates of passive diffusion of ions across the tubular wall. Secondly, the reabsorption of sodium and chloride, the most abundant solutes in the filtrate, establishes osmotic gradients across the tubular epithelium that cause the passive reabsorption of water. Thirdly, the reabsorption of water from the tubular fluid in turn increases the concentrations of other substances in the remaining fluid and thus modifies the chemical gradients for passive diffusion of these substances. A prime example of such a substance is urea. Most of the filtered urea is reabsorbed passively. The chemical gradient for net passive diffusion out of the tubule is established by water reabsorption, which in turn, is dependent on active salt reabsorption. In addition, the electrochemical gradient for Na itself may provide the energy required for transport of other substances. For example, the first step in reabsorption of glucose and amino acids from the tubular fluid involves their transport across the luminal membrane of tubular cells into the cell. The transport process in the membrane for the organic molecule requires the presence of Na. It transfers both Na and the organic molecule through the membrane together, and the rate of transport is dependent on the electrochemical gradient for Na. The mechanism responsible for this cotransport is called a symport.

The transport of solutes in response to the electrochemical gradients that result from salt and water transport requires no direct utilization of metabolic energy. However, such energy is expended in the establishment and maintenance of these gradients by the active transport mechanisms for salt. Thus, inhibition or stimulation of these mechanisms by drugs, hormones, or other factors accomplishes far more than just an alteration in the rate of salt reabsorption.

There are many other examples of interdependence among the tubular transport processes. Despite this, the nephron can selectively change the excretion rate of many substances within certain limits without seriously interrupting the function of other tubular processes.

Each nephron can operate independently of its neighbors in many respects. This is not true for at least two important processes, the osmotic concentration of the urine and urea excretion, as shall be described later. All nephrons are generally assumed to function alike qualitatively. However, since they differ in length, it is believed that there are quantitative differences in their functional capacity. Also, it is usually considered that all nephrons function continually to some degree, but the GFR and the volume reabsorbed per unit time may change in any one nephron or groups of nephrons without large changes in the GFR for the entire kidney.

In considering the general features of the function of the individual nephron segments, it is useful to compare and contrast the functions of the proximal tubule with the "distal nephron." The latter term includes all the remaining segments, the loop of Henle, the distal tubule, and the collecting tubule. The greater fraction of the filtrate (60 to 70%) is reabsorbed in the proximal tubule. Because of the high hydraulic conductance or water permeability and high electrical or ionic conductance of the tubular epithelium, this reabsorption takes place without any change in the osmotic and sodium concentrations of the filtrate and with only relatively minor changes in the concentration of other electrolytes. Thus, in terms of water and most electrolytes, "bulk" reabsorption of the filtrate occurs in the proximal tubule with little change in the composition of the tubular fluid. Importantly, this is not true for organic substances. Almost all transport of organic substances, with the major exception of urea, occurs in the proximal tubule. Glucose and most amino acids are almost totally reabsorbed and essentially disappear from the proximal tubular fluid. Secretion of other organic compounds, some naturally occurring, such as urate, and many foreign to the body, such as penicillin, also takes place here. Most of the reabsorption that occurs in the proximal tubule is powered by active Na transport and, to a lesser extent, by active bicarbonate reabsorption. Transfer of the reabsorbate from the tubular lumen to the circulation is assisted by the favorable balance of colloid osmotic pressure and hydrostatic pressure within the peritubular capillaries that surround the tubules.

In the "distal nephron" the hydraulic conductance and ionic conductance vary along the length of the segments and also vary in response to hormonal influence. Generally, both conductances are lower than in the proximal tubule. Thus, the osmotic and electrolyte concentrations vary widely along the distal nephron and vary widely in time in response to changes in plasma levels of antidiuretic hormone and aldosterone. The loop of Henle of juxtamedullary nephrons and the collecting tubules pass through the medulla. Transport by these structures, together with the countercurrent flow of tubular fluid through the loop of Henle and of blood through the vasa recta, drastically alters the extracellular environment of that tissue from that which prevails in the cortex and in the rest of the body. In turn, that unique extracellular environment in the medulla exerts a powerful influence on the composition of tubular fluid. Active sodium transport is the major generating force for reabsorption of salt, water, and urea in the distal nephron. Potassium reabsorption and potassium and hydrogen secretion occur in various segments. The only major organic substances that are transported in the distal nephron are urea and ammonia.

We can contrast then the bulk reabsorption of water and electrolytes in the proximal tubule, where the proportion of electrolyte reabsorbed to water reabsorbed is relatively fixed, to the reabsorption that occurs in the distal nephron where the reabsorption of electrolytes and water can occur in widely varying proportions. Consequently, the osmotic concentration of the final urine may vary from as low as 40 to 50 mOsm/kg H_2O to as high as 1400 mOsm/kg H_2O, and the concentration of the various electrolytes can be much higher or much lower than their plasma concentration.

It is important to remember that the concentration of any one substance in the final urine depends not only on the rate of transport of that substance by the nephron, but also on the rate of water reabsorption. In order to determine how the rate of transport of a particular substance changes in various circumstances, one must consider the rate of excretion of that substance rather than its concentration. Moreover, because the intake of various substances, and particularly the intake of water by a normal individual, varies over a wide range, it is a fallacy to consider that there is a "normal" urine composition.

BIBLIOGRAPHY

Historical:

Austin, J. H., Stillman, E., and Van Slyke, D. D.: Factors governing the excretion rate of urea. J. Biol. Chem., 46:91, 1921.

Barber, M. A.: A New Method of Isolating Micro-Organisms. J. Kans. Med. Soc., 4:487, 1904.

Bellini, L., and Borelli, J. A.: De Structura Renum, Observatio Anatomica. 2nd ed. Pisa, S. Paulli, 1664.

Bowman, W.: On the structure and use of the Malpighian bodies of the kidney, with observations on the circulation through that gland. Philos. Trans. Roy. Soc., 132:57, 1842.

Bronk, D. W.: Alfred Newton Richards (1876-1966). Perspect. Biol. Med. 19:413, 1976.

Cushny, A. R.: The Secretion of the Urine. London, Longmans, Green and Co., 1917.

Heidenhain, R.: Mikroskopische Beiträge zur Anatomie und Physiologie der Nieren. Arch. Mikr. Anat., 10:1, 1874.

Heidenhain, R., and Neisser, A.: Versuche über den Vorgang der Harnabsonderung. Pflügers Arch ges Physiol., 9:1, 1874.

Jolliffe, N., Shannon, J. A., and Smith, H. W.: Excretion of urine in dog; use of non-metabolized sugars in measurement of glomerular filtrate. Am. J. Physiol., 101:301, 1932.

Ludwig, C.: Beiträge zur Lehre vom Mechanismus der Harnesecretion. Marburg, Elwert, 1843.

Malpighi, M.: Malpighi's "Concerning the structure of kidneys." Translated by J. M. Hayman, Jr., Ann. Med. Hist., 7:242, 1925.

Marshall, E. K., Jr., and Vickers, J. L.: The mechanism of elimination of phenolsulpho-nephthalen by the kidney—a proof of secretion by the convoluted tubules. Bull. Johns Hopkins Hosp., 34:1, 1923.

Rehberg, P. B.: Studies on kidney function. 1. The rate of filtration and reabsorption in the human kidney. Biochem. J., 20:447, 1926.

Richards, A. N.: Methods and Results of Direct Investigations of the Functions of the Kidney. Baltimore, Williams and Wilkins, 1929.

Richards, A. N.: Processes of urine formation. The Croonian Lecture. Proc. Roy. Soc. B, 126:398, 1938.

Smith, Homer W.: Lectures on the Kidney. Lawrence, Univ. of Kansas, 1943.

Smith, Homer W.: Renal Physiology. In Circulation of the Blood, Men and Ideas. Edited by A. P. Fishman, and D. W. Richards. New York, Oxford Univ. Press, 1964.

Wearn, J. T.: Composition of glomerular urine with conclusive evidence of reabsorption in the renal tubules. Physiologist, 23:1, 1980.

Wearn, J. T., and Richards, A. N.: Observations on the composition of glomerular urine, with particular reference to the problem of reabsorption in the renal tubules. Am. J. Physiol., 71:209, 1924.

Anatomic:

Rouiller, C.: General Anatomy and Histology of the Kidney. In The Kidney, Vol. 1. Edited by C. Rouiller, and A. F. Muller, New York, Academic Press, 1969.

Tisher, C. C.: Anatomy of the Kidney. *In* The Kidney, 2nd ed. Vol. 1. Edited by B. M. Brenner, and F. C. Rector, Jr. Philadelphia, W. B. Saunders Co. 1981.

Functional:

Berliner, R. W., and Giebisch, G.: Body Fluids and the Excretion of the Urine. *In* Best and Taylor's Physiological Basis of Medical Practice. 10th ed. Edited by J. R. Brobeck, Baltimore, Williams and Wilkins, 1979.
Lassiter, W. E., and Gottschalk, C. W.: The Kidney and Body Fluids. *In* Medical Physiology. 13th Ed. Edited by V. B. Mountcastle, St. Louis, C. V. Mosby, 1974.
Pitts, R. F.: Physiology of the Kidney and Body Fluids. 3rd ed. Chicago, Year Book Medical Publishers, 1974.
Wesson, L. G. Jr.: Physiology of the Human Kidney. New York, Grune and Stratton, 1969.

CHAPTER 3

Measurement of Renal Function

Measurement of the varied functions of the kidney depends almost entirely on the application of the principle of conservation. For substances that are not synthesized or metabolized by renal tissue, the amount entering the kidney via the renal artery equals the amount leaving in the renal vein and ureter. Similarly, the amount entering the nephrons by filtration or secretion equals the amount leaving by reabsorption or excretion. The use of this principle provides the means for indirectly measuring renal blood flow, glomerular filtration rate, and the rates of tubular reabsorption and secretion of various substances.

RENAL PLASMA FLOW

Renal plasma flow can be determined by the principle of conservation and the use of a substance that is not synthesized or metabolized by the kidney. The amount of such a substance entering the kidney per unit time via the renal artery equals the arterial plasma flow rate (RPF^a) times the concentration in the arterial plasma (P_s^a). In the steady state, that same amount leaves the kidney at the same rate in the urine and in the renal venous blood. The rate of exit in the urine equals the urine concentration of the substance (U_s) times the urine flow rate ($\dot{V}$). The rate of exit in the venous blood equals the renal venous plasma flow (RPF^v) times the concentration in the renal venous plasma (P_s^{rv}). Therefore:

$$RPF^a \times P_s^a = (RPF^v \times P_s^{rv}) + U_s\dot{V}$$

The plasma flow in the renal vein is slightly smaller than that in the artery, since the urine volume is extracted from the plasma. Usually, this difference is so small (1/660) that it is ignored and the above equation is simplified to:

$$RPF\,(P_s^a - P_s^{rv}) = U_s\dot{V}\text{ and}$$

$$RPF = \frac{U_s\dot{V}}{P_s^a - P_s^{rv}} \qquad \text{(ml/min)}$$

In principle, any substance that is not metabolized or synthesized by the kidney could be used to measure RPF. Practically, an accurate measure cannot be obtained unless the kidney excretes a substantial amount and there is a significant difference between the arterial and renal venous concentrations.

The difficulty of obtaining renal venous plasma samples limits the usefulness of this approach to measuring RPF. However, it has been found that the tubular secretory system for para-aminohippurate (PAH) is so efficient that at low plasma concentrations it removes 90% or more of the PAH from the plasma as it flows through the kidney. Actually, the proximal tubules may remove almost all the PAH in the plasma that perfuses them. The other 10% may be in plasma that perfuses medullary and nontubular tissues. So, for determining plasma flow to tubular tissue, P_{PAH}^{rv} is considered to equal zero and the equation becomes

$$RPF = \frac{U_{PAH}\dot{V}}{P_{PAH}} \qquad \text{(ml/min)}$$

The plasma flow determined in this manner is considered to be the effective renal plasma flow (ERPF), that is, the plasma perfusing functional tubular tissue, rather than the total renal plasma flow. This is a common assumption, but is probably not valid since blood perfusing the medulla may not have its PAH removed.

The renal blood flow may be calculated from measurement of the RPF and the hematocrit as follows:

$$RBF = RPF + (RBF \times Hct)$$

$$RBF\,(1 - Hct) = RPF$$

$$RBF = \frac{RPF}{1 - Hct}$$

GLOMERULAR FILTRATION RATE

The total plasma volume filtered by the glomeruli per unit time (GFR) can be measured by the use of the conservation principle and a substance that is freely filtered but is not reabsorbed or secreted to a significant extent, so that the amount excreted equals the amount filtered. The substance must also have no effect on renal function. One such substance is inulin, a fructose polysaccharide with a molecular weight of approximately 5000.

The amount of inulin filtered per unit time by the glomeruli equals the volume of plasma filtered (GFR) times the plasma concentration (P_{in}) (Fig. 3-1). The amount exiting from the ureter per unit time equals the urine volume per unit time ($\dot{V}$) times the urine concentration (U_{in}). Since the tubular cells do not add or remove inulin from the filtrate to an appreciable extent, the amount entering the nephrons equals the amount exiting within experimental error thus:

$$\text{GFR} \times P_{in} = U_{in}\dot{V}$$

Plasma and urine concentrations and urine volume can be measured, so

$$\text{GFR} = \frac{U_{in}\dot{V}}{P_{in}} \qquad \text{(ml/min)}$$

TUBULAR TRANSPORT

With the use of a measurement of GFR and the conservation principle, the rate of tubular reabsorption of substances from the filtrate or the rate of tubular secretion of substances into the tubular fluid can be measured. Most substances handled by the kidney are freely filterable, so the amount filtered per unit time equals the GFR times the plasma concen-

MEASUREMENT OF FILTRATION

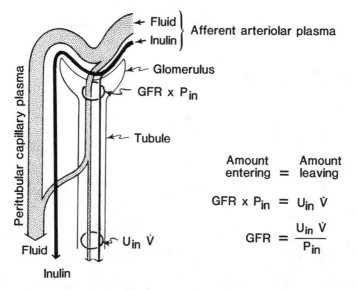

Figure 3-1. Measurement of filtration. Fluid and solute, which of course are thoroughly mixed in the circulation and within the tubule, are shown separately here for purposes of illustration. The amounts referred to are the amounts of solute entering and leaving the nephron.

tration of the substance (P_s). For substances reabsorbed by the tubular cells (Fig. 3-2), the amount entering the tubules by filtration equals the amount transported out of the tubules (T) plus the amount exiting into the ureter, that is:

$$\text{GFR} \times P_s = T + U_s\dot{V} \text{ and}$$

$$(\text{GFR} \times P_s) - U_s\dot{V} = T \qquad \text{(mg/min)}$$

For substances secreted by the tubular cells, the amount entering the nephrons equals the amount filtered plus the amount secreted or transported (T) into the tubule (Fig. 3-3). This sum is equal to the amount excreted:

$$(\text{GFR} \times P_s) + T = U_s\dot{V} \text{ and}$$

$$T = U_s\dot{V} - (\text{GFR} \times P_s) \qquad \text{(mg/min)}$$

THE CONCEPT OF CLEARANCE

To excrete a substance such as inulin, the kidney filters a large volume of plasma containing inulin, then the tubular cells reabsorb almost all of this fluid, returning it to the circulation without inulin, which remains behind and is excreted in the urine. By this process, the kidney has "cleared" a volume of plasma, equivalent to the volume of the filtrate,

MEASUREMENT OF REABSORPTION

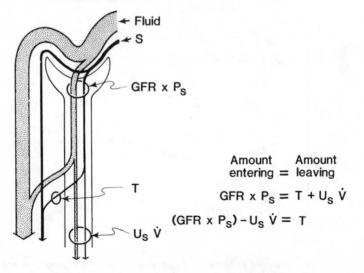

Figure 3-2. Measurement of reabsorption. T equals the amount of solute transported from the tubular fluid into the peritubular capillary plasma.

MEASUREMENT OF SECRETION

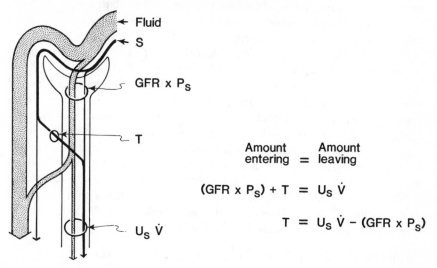

$$(GFR \times P_S) + T = U_S \dot{V}$$

$$T = U_S \dot{V} - (GFR \times P_S)$$

Figure 3-3. Measurement of secretion. T equals the amount of solute transported into the tubule from the peritubular capillary plasma.

of the inulin contained within it. Thus the volume of plasma cleared of inulin per unit time is as follows:

$$C_{in} = GFR = \frac{U_{in}\dot{V}}{P_{in}} \qquad (ml/min)$$

C_{in} is a virtual volume, the smallest volume of plasma sufficient to account for the amount of inulin excreted per unit time.

For reabsorbed substances, the apparent volume of plasma cleared of the substance is smaller than the filtered volume since some of the substance is returned to the plasma from the filtrate by the tubular cells. Nevertheless, the amount excreted ($U_s\dot{V}$) can be considered to have been contained in a virtual volume of plasma (C_s) at the plasma concentration:

$$C_s = \frac{U_s\dot{V}}{P_s} \qquad (ml/min)$$

For substances that are reabsorbed, the apparent clearance (C_s) is less than the clearance of inulin (C_{in}).

For substances that are filtered and secreted but not reabsorbed to a significant extent, the amount excreted exceeds the amount filtered. The volume of plasma cleared of the substance is larger than the glomerular filtrate or the clearance of inulin, because the tubular cells are also removing the substance from plasma in the peritubular capillaries. Still, the amount of the substance excreted was contained initially in a certain volume of plasma at the plasma concentration. The standard clearance equation given above can be used to calculate the apparent volume of plasma that was cleared by both filtration and secretion.

To summarize, clearance may be defined as the virtual volume of plasma that the kidney has cleared of a substance per unit time or, to state it another way, clearance is the virtual volume of plasma that contained the mass of a substance that the kidney excreted in a unit of time. For a substance that is neither reabsorbed nor secreted and meets the other criteria given, the clearance rate equals the GFR. From here on the terms GFR and C_{in} will be used interchangeably. For a substance that is filtered and reabsorbed, $C_s < C_{in}$ and for a substance that is filtered and secreted, $C_s > C_{in}$. These facts are used experimentally to determine how substances are handled by the kidney.

Effect of Changes in Plasma Concentration On Clearance Rates

For substances that are filtered only, the amount of the substance filtered and excreted will increase as the plasma concentration rises, but the volume of fluid filtered will not change; thus the volume of fluid cleared will not change (A in Fig. 3-4). However, the transport processes for substances that are reabsorbed or secreted usually can handle only limited amounts of the substances and this affects the clearance rates. As the plasma concentration of a reabsorbed substance rises and the amount filtered increases, the transport process becomes saturated and a greater fraction of the filtered amount escapes reabsorption and is excreted. Because of this, a larger fraction of the filtered fluid is returned to the circulation cleared of the substance (B in Fig. 3-4). As the plasma concentration of a secreted substance increases and the transport process becomes saturated, a smaller fraction of the total amount in the blood flowing past the tubular cells is secreted into the tubules and the volume of plasma cleared of the substances falls (C in Fig. 3-4).

An example of the changes that occur when the plasma concentration of a reabsorbed substance such as glucose is increased is illustrated in Figure 3-5. At the normal plasma level (0.8 to 1.0 mg/ml), all filtered glucose is reabsorbed (Fig. 3-5A) and $C_G = 0$ (Fig. 3-5B). As the plasma concentration rises (1 to 2 mg/ml), the amount filtered per unit time, and thus the amount presented for reabsorption, rises. The rate of reabsorption increases initially, no glucose is excreted and C_G still equals zero. If the plasma concentration continues to increase (>3 mg/ml), the maximum transport rate (Tm_G) is reached. As the amount filtered continues to rise above that point, there is no further increase in reabsorption, the excess is excreted in increasing amounts, and the volume of plasma cleared of glucose increases and approaches the volume filtered.

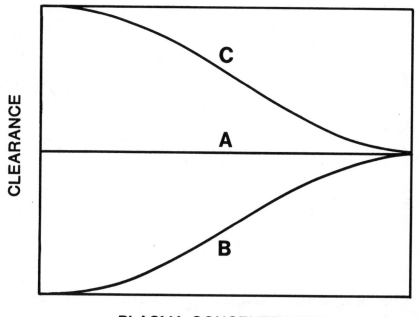

PLASMA CONCENTRATION

Figure 3-4.   The effect of changes in concentration of various solutes in plasma on their clearance from plasma. A is a substance that is filtered but not reabsorbed or secreted, such as inulin. B is a substance that is filtered and reabsorbed, such as glucose. C is a substance that is filtered and secreted, such as PAH.

The changes that follow an increase in the concentration of a secreted substance such as PAH are illustrated in Figure 3-6. At low plasma concentrations, almost all PAH is removed from the blood flowing through the kidney by the processes of filtration and secretion, and the clearance rate approximately equals the RPF. Initially, as the plasma concentration increases (up to ~0.1 mg/ml), the secretory mechanism continues to transport almost all the PAH presented to it, the amount secreted increases, and almost all the plasma is still cleared of PAH. However, when the plasma concentration increases beyond the point at which the transport system becomes saturated, some of the PAH escapes secretion and the volume of plasma cleared of PAH falls.

TUBULAR TRANSPORT MAXIMA

The measurement of the maximum rate of transport (Tm) for a substance is sometimes useful in clinical experiments to determine the amount of functional tubular tissue. The criteria for accurate measurement of Tm are as follows: (1) Plasma levels must be high enough to

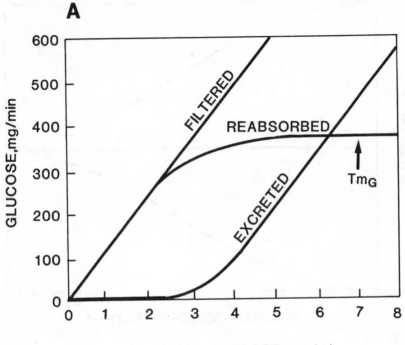

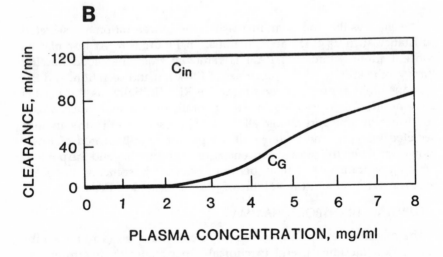

Figure 3-5. The effect of changes in the plasma concentration of glucose on its rates of filtration, reabsorption, excretion, and clearance.

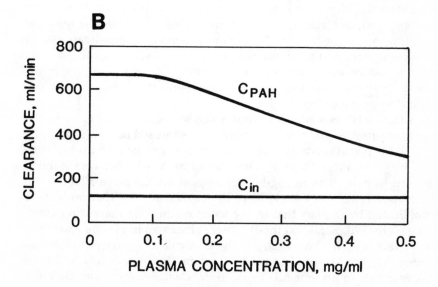

Figure 3-6. The effect of changes in the plasma concentration of PAH on its rates of filtration, secretion, excretion, and clearance.

saturate the transport system. (2) Two consecutive clearance determinations must be made in which the plasma concentration rises, but the calculated amount of substance transported does not. This ensures that the tubular maximum has been reached.

CLINICAL MEASUREMENT OF RENAL FUNCTION

GFR and RPF

The clearance of inulin is the most accurate measure of GFR available. However, several factors limit the use of inulin clearance in the common clinical situation. An intravenous injection followed by a constant infusion is required. Complete emptying of the bladder is necessary before the beginning of the clearance period, in order to remove all urine not containing inulin, and again at the end of the period, in order to obtain all urine produced during the period. The urine flow must be high so that enough urine may be obtained in a short period of time to permit analysis and to reduce possible errors introduced by urine remaining in the bladder at the beginning and end of the clearance period. These requirements often cannot be met in a patient with compromised renal function.

The use of creatinine clearance as a measure of GFR overcomes many of these practical problems, but introduces others. Creatinine (molecular weight = 113) is an end product of protein metabolism. It is always present in the blood, and its concentration (0.5 to 1.2 mg/dl) remains relatively constant over a 24-hour period. This eliminates the need for an intravenous infusion, and therefore a clearance period can extend over a long period of time, usually 24 hours, so that adequate amounts of urine can be obtained and the problem of bladder emptying minimized. Only one blood sample is needed, and it can be taken at any point during the collection period.

Creatinine is freely filtered, but it is also secreted into the urine by the proximal tubular epithelium. If creatinine is infused into an individual to raise the plasma concentration, its clearance exceeds the inulin clearance by 10 to 40%. There is some doubt as to whether creatinine is secreted in more than negligible amounts at normal plasma levels, but the preponderance of the evidence indicates that it is. This problem is complicated by the fact that in the usual method for measuring creatinine (Folin Wu picrate method), other substances in plasma react with the picrate reagent. The nature of these so-called "noncreatinine chromogens" is not known, but evidently their clearance is low and their concentration in urine is nil. Thus, in the clearance equation, $U_{cr}\dot{V}/P_{cr}$, the value of the denominator is raised by the presence of these chromogens, and the value of the numerator is presumably raised by tubular secretion of true creatinine. These two factors partially cancel each other and the net result is that the clearance approximates the GFR.

In using creatinine clearance to measure GFR, the fact that creatinine is secreted should be kept in mind. It is possible that falsely high clearance values may be obtained in patients with poor glomerular function but with good blood flow and tubular function. Conversely, certain drugs (organic cations such as cimetidine and trimethoprim) inhibit tubular secretion of creatinine causing the apparent creatinine clearance to decrease. In addition, one must have some knowledge of the method used to determine creatinine concentrations. The proportion of true creatinine concentration to noncreatinine chromogen in plasma changes when glomerular filtration drops, and the true plasma creatinine concentration rises as a result of reduced excretion.

All the difficulties involved in measuring inulin clearance in patients are also encountered in measuring PAH clearance. In addition, a compromised or diseased kidney may not be extracting 90% of the PAH from the plasma flowing through it, so renal venous blood samples must be obtained in order to measure RPF accurately. Consequently, other means of assessing RPF have been developed. In general, these methods are only semiquantitative, but are much more easily applied to patients.

In one of these methods, a substance secreted by tubular cells is labelled with a radioactive isotope (commonly ^{131}I) and given as a single intravenous injection. An isotope counter is placed over the kidney and the amount of isotope appearing in that region of the body is measured. Following the injection, the isotope rapidly accumulates in the normal kidney as the tubules remove the substance from the plasma. After reaching a peak, the amount of isotope present falls at a somewhat slower rate as it is excreted in the urine. In other methods, the rate of disappearance of the same type of substance from the circulating plasma is measured after a single injection. This can be done by sequentially removing aliquots of blood and measuring the radioactivity present or by placing a counter over the head and measuring the radioactivity circulating through the head. The rate at which this substance disappears from the blood is largely determined by the rate at which the kidney clears it from the circulating plasma.

Use of Concentration Ratios

Various types of concentration ratios are often used in assessing tubular function in patients. Since they do not require measurement of the urine flow rate, long periods of urine collection are not necessary. For instance, the concentration in the urine of a substance, which, like inulin, is not transported by the tubular epithelium, changes from the plasma concentration only as water is reabsorbed. Thus the ratio U_{in}/P_{in} serves as an index of the degree of water reabsorption. For example, if U_{in}/P_{in} equals 2, 50% of the filtered water has been reabsorbed; if the ratio equals 4, 75% has been reabsorbed and so on. Clinically, it is more practical to use the creatinine concentration ratio, U_{cr}/P_{cr} for this purpose.

One of the most important functions of tubular cells is the active reabsorption of Na. In the distal sections of the nephron, this results in a fall in the tubular fluid Na concentration. Therefore, in certain circumstances, the ratio U_{Na}/P_{Na} can be used as a measure of the ability of these distal sections to establish and maintain a concentration gradient for Na across the tubular wall. Both the Na ratio and the creatinine ratio can be useful in assessing the degree of tubular damage in a kidney that has undergone a period of acute injury.

Since the urine concentrations of substances like Na, K, urea, and uric acid are a function not only of tubular transport but also of the reabsorption of water, the use of a double ratio is often more practical:

$$\frac{U_s/P_s}{U_{cr}/P_{cr}}$$

(The mnemonic that results is such that no student should ever forget the ratio.) Factoring the concentration ratio of a transported substance by the ratio for creatinine corrects for the effect of water reabsorption and thus measures only the degree of transport of the substance. This double ratio is derived from the ratio of the clearance rates of the two substances and measures the fractional excretion rate of the substance (FE_s).

$$FE_s = \frac{C_s}{C_{cr}} = \frac{U_s\dot{V}/P_s}{U_{cr}\dot{V}/P_{cr}} = \frac{U_s/P_s}{U_{cr}/P_{cr}}$$

The fractional reabsorption rate, FR_s is equal to $1 - FE_s$. FE_s and FR_s are usually multiplied by 100 to give the percent of the filtered amount of the substance that is either absorbed or excreted.

Almost all substances normally found in the filtrate are only reabsorbed by the tubules or, as is true of uric acid, reabsorbed in greater amounts than are secreted. Thus FE_s is usually less than one and FR_s is a positive value. The only notable exceptions to this are potassium and ammonium. For ammonium, secretion always exceeds reabsorption, FE_{NH_3} is greater than one, and calculation of FR_{NH_3} has no meaning. For potassium, the amount reabsorbed usually exceeds the amount secreted and FE_K is usually less than one. However, in certain physiologic situations and in patients with advanced renal disease in which GFR is greatly reduced, secretion may predominate and FE_K may exceed one or 100%. Normal values for FR_s are listed in Table 2-1.

Utility of Plasma Creatinine Measurement in Chronic Patients

The major factor that alters the plasma creatinine concentration over periods of days, months, or years is the GFR. Normally, the rate of filtration of creatinine $(P_{cr} \cdot GFR)$ and the rate of excretion $(U_{cr}\dot{V})$ equals the rate of production of creatinine. The rate of production does not vary to an appreciable extent in an individual over a period of time, so when GFR is stable, P_{cr} is also stable. If GFR is reduced, the rate of filtration of creatinine is momentarily reduced. This causes P_{cr} to rise until the product ($P_{cr} \cdot$ GFR) returns to its previous level, and once again, the rate of excretion equals the rate of production. If one considers the clearance equation $C_{cr} = $ GFR $ = U_{cr}\dot{V}/P_{cr}$, it is apparent that since $U_{cr}\dot{V}$ is a constant, $1/P_{cr}$ varies as the GFR varies. Measurement of P_{cr} and calculation of the reciprocal in a patient with chronic disease, with time, will serve as an indication of the changes in glomerular function, as Figure 3-7 illustrates. If the disease process is accelerated, the reciprocal will fall at an increased rate; if treatment halts the progression of the disease, the reciprocal will stabilize.

As an example, consider a patient in the initial stages of glomerulonephritis. The rate of production and excretion of creatinine equals 1440 mg/day. Initially, the P_{cr} is 1.0 mg/dl.

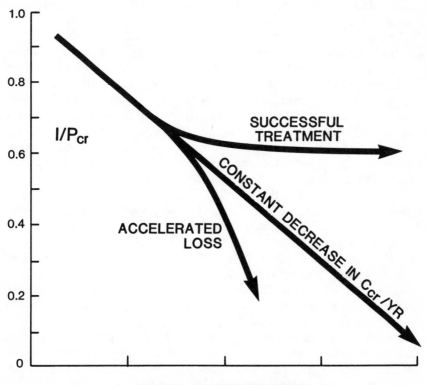

Figure 3-7. Use of the reciprocal of plasma creatinine concentration, $1/P_{cr}$, to follow the progress of glomerular disease in a patient.

$$GFR = \frac{1440 \text{ mg/day} \times 1 \text{ day/1440 min}}{1 \text{ mg/dl} \times 1 \text{ dl/100 ml}} = \frac{1 \text{ mg/min}}{.01 \text{ mg/ml}} = 100 \text{ ml/min}$$

One year later, it is found that P_{cr} now equals 1.5 mg/dl in this patient. Assuming that the rate of production and excretion of creatinine has not changed, the calculation above indicates the GFR has been reduced 33%. Initially, $1/P_{cr}$ equalled 1; now it equals 0.67. Two years later $P_{cr} = 3.0$, $1/P_{cr} = 0.33$, indicating that the patient has lost 67% of his glomerular function. Obviously, there has been a steady progression of the disease.

METHODS FOR EXPERIMENTAL INVESTIGATION

The method most commonly used to study renal function both clinically and experimentally is the clearance method described earlier. In general, this method, which was developed by Homer Smith and his co-workers, allows quantitative measurement of the filtration rate and the rates of transport of substances by the entire kidney. However, information on the function of a particular segment of the nephron cannot be obtained by this method except by indirect means.

The micropuncture technique, developed initially by A. N. Richards and his associates, is the most versatile method for studying renal function and has provided the most detailed information of cellular function in certain segments of the nephron. Basically, the technique involves the puncture of individual tubular segments on the surface of an exposed kidney with micropipets, the withdrawal of small tubular fluid samples for quantitative analysis, and subsequent localization of the puncture site along the length of the nephron. The technique can be modified to permit study of the electrical properties of tubular epithelium with the use of microelectrodes. Moreover, segments of the nephron may be perfused with artificial fluids, which can be subsequently withdrawn for chemical analysis. It is also possible to puncture and perfuse the capillary bed supplying the tubular segment under study.

Micropuncture is a fairly arduous technique because the small diameter of the nephron requires the use of pipets with a tip diameter of less than 20 microns and because only a few nanoliters (10^{-9} L) of fluid can be collected for analysis. The technique can be used to study only those tubular segments that appear on the surface of the cortex and, in certain animals, in the tip of the papilla.

A more limited method is that of stop flow analysis. An animal is made to diurese by intravenous infusion of a poorly reabsorbed solute such as mannitol and the ureter of one kidney is exposed and catheterized. After the urine flow has stabilized at a high level, the catheter is clamped for a short time (<15 min). Since the poorly reabsorbed solute inhibits water reabsorption, the pressure within the nephron rapidly increases and glomerular filtration is greatly reduced. In this way, the various transport mechanisms are given a long period of time in which to alter the concentration of substances in the columns of tubular fluid trapped in the nephrons. When the clamp is released, the columns of fluid moving out of the nephrons, in effect, are serially sectioned by the collection of serial urine samples. If inulin is injected intravenously during the occlusion period, its appearance late in the serial samples signals the entry of fluid that was filtered after the occlusion. The concentration profiles of Na and PAH in the serial samples serve to identify the tubular sites of the samples, since the Na concentration can be reduced to low levels only in the distal sections of the nephrons and the concentration of PAH is increased by secretion only in the proximal tubule. This technique allows a closer study of separate parts of the nephrons than does the clearance method and is technically easier than the micropuncture method. However, it cannot approach the nephron as directly as the micropuncture technique and the data that can be obtained are much more limited and sometimes difficult to quantify.

A versatile technique for perfusing isolated fragments of the nephron has been developed more recently. A segment of the nephron is dissected free of surrounding tissue and placed in a chamber on the stage of an inverted microscope. Micropipets are positioned at each end of the segment and fluid is perfused through the segment and collected. With this technique, the composition of both the perfusion fluid and the fluid surrounding the nephron segment can be precisely controlled. Nephron segments not accessible for micropuncture can be studied as well. The method is technically demanding, and since the segments studied are totally separated from other structures in the kidney, caution must be exerted in using the results to interpret what occurs in the intact kidney.

The study of transport in other epithelial tissues has also provided a wealth of information that can be applied to renal physiology. Frog skin and the urinary bladder of the toad, for instance, both actively transport Na from pond water or urine into the blood and respond to hormones that also affect renal function. Experimental techniques for studying these tissues are relatively simple. Basic information on the mechanism of action of antidiuretic hormone and aldosterone and on the properties of the Na transport system has been obtained from these studies.

Appendix to Chapter 3

A TYPICAL CLEARANCE EXPERIMENT

A. Object: To measure GFR, RPF, Tm_G and Tm_{PAH}
B. Plan:
    1. GFR will be measured by determining the clearance of inulin.
    2. Renal plasma flow will be measured by determining the clearance of PAH. This will be done while the plasma level of PAH is maintained at a low level, so that the transport maximum for PAH will not be reached and the renal venous blood concentration of PAH will be negligible. These conditions must be met if the clearance of PAH is to equal the effective renal plasma flow.
    3. To measure the transport maxima for glucose and PAH, the plasma level of these two substances will later be raised in steps until the tubular transport mechanisms for these two substances are saturated so that glucose appears in the urine and PAH appears in larger amounts in the renal venous blood. To assure that the tubular mechanisms are saturated, successive clearance periods will be performed while the plasma level is raised. When the calculated reabsorptive rate for glucose and the secretory rate for PAH do not increase from one clearance period to the next while the plasma level does increase, we can be assured that more glucose and PAH are being presented to the transport mechanisms than they can handle. Then we can assume that the mechanisms are transporting at their maximum rate.
C. Procedure:
    1. Inject intravenously a priming dose of inulin and PAH to bring the plasma level of the two compounds to a suitable point.
    2. Start a constant infusion of inulin and PAH in order to replace what is excreted and thus keep the plasma level constant.
    3. Place a catheter through the urethra to the bladder.
    4. Empty bladder.
    5. Begin a 10-minute urine collection period (clearance period).
    6. Collect blood samples at beginning and end of collection period.
    7. Immediately repeat steps 5 and 6 above.
    8. Raise plasma concentration of glucose and PAH in steps. After each increase, perform a 10-minute clearance period as in steps 5 and 6.

9. Measure urine and plasma concentration of inulin, glucose, and PAH. Measure urine volume and calculate urine flow in ml per min for each collection.

D. Protocol and Data Record

TIME	P_{IN} mg/ml	P_G mg/ml	P_{PAH} mg/ml	$\dot{V}$ ml/min	U_{IN} mg/ml	U_G mg/ml	U_{PAH} mg/ml
0 min	— Inject priming dose of inulin and PAH intravenously						

0 min Inject priming dose of inulin and PAH intravenously
2 min Begin constant infusion of inulin and PAH
15 min Urethra catheterized
29 min Empty bladder
30 min Begin first urine collection period and collect blood sample
  1.10 0.9 0.052 Hematocrit—43%
40 min End first urine collection period, begin second and collect blood sample
  1.20 0.88 0.054 1.9 64 0 17.3
50 min End second urine collection period and collect blood sample
  1.25 0.93 0.055 1.8 78 0 18.5
  Hematocrit—42%
52 min Begin infusion of glucose and increased amount of PAH
75 min Begin third clearance period and collect blood sample
  1.15 1.5 0.090
85 min End third clearance period and collect blood sample
  1.12 1.6 0.095 1.7 72 0 34
87 min Increase infusion rate of glucose and PAH
115 min Begin fourth clearance period and collect blood sample
  1.30 2.5 0.15
125 min End fourth clearance period and collect blood sample
  1.16 2.6 0.16 2.3 56 20 40
127 min Increase infusion rate of glucose and PAH
155 min Begin fifth clearance period and collect blood sample
  1.10 3.5 0.25
165 min End fifth clearance period and collect blood sample
  1.18 3.6 0.26 2.7 48 38 41
167 min Increase infusion rate of glucose and PAH
195 min Begin sixth clearance period and collect blood sample
  1.2 4.2 0.30
205 min End sixth clearance period and collect blood sample
  1.14 4.3 0.32 3.0 46 44 39
207 min Increase infusion rate of glucose and PAH
235 min Begin seventh clearance period and collect blood sample
  1.12 4.8 0.38
245 min End seventh period and collect blood sample
  1.16 4.9 0.40 3.2 39 50 39
247 min Stop infusions.

PROBLEMS

1. Calculate the subject's GFR for the first and last clearance periods. (In all calculations, the plasma concentrations obtained at the beginning and end of a clearance period should be averaged and the average value used in your calculations for the period.)
2. Using the date from the *appropriate* clearance periods, calculate the subject's RPF, RBF, Tm_G and Tm_{PAH}.
3. Why does the clearance of glucose change as the plasma concentration rises? What other substances would follow a similar pattern? Why does the clearance of PAH change as the plasma concentration rises? What other substances would follow a similar pattern?
4. The following values were determined in a subject who was in sodium and water "balance": plasma creatinine, 1.1 mg/dl; urine creatinine, 146 mg/dl; and urine volume, 1280 ml per 24 hours. (a) Calculate the rate of creatinine clearance. (b) What fraction of the plasma filtered by the glomeruli was excreted? (c) What fraction of the filtered plasma was reabsorbed?
5. For the following urine-to-plasma creatinine ratios, calculate the fractional excretion and the fractional reabsorption of filtered plasma.

U/P creatinine
   a.   2.00
   b.   4.75
   c.   34.20
   d.   107
   e.   420

6. The following values were obtained from a patient who was in salt and water balance.

	Creatinine mg/dl	Sodium mEq/L	Urate mg/dl	Volume
Plasma	0.9	140	6.8	
Urine	110	88	84	890 ml/24 hours

Calculate (a) the creatinine clearance, (b) the rate of sodium filtration, (c) the rate of sodium excretion, (d) the fractional excretion and reabsorption of sodium, and (e) the fractional excretion of urate.

7. A patient with chronic, slowly progressive renal failure was found to have the following laboratory values. Calculate (a) the creatinine clearance and (b) the fractional excretion of Na, K, PO_4. How do you explain the unusually high FE_K value?

	Creatinine mg/dl	Sodium mEq/L	Potassium mEq/L	Phosphate mg/dl	Volume
Plasma	8.5	135	4.9	7.0	—
Urine	54	40	46	17.0	1800 ml/day

8. Compare and contrast the following for the patients described in problems 6 and 7: (a) $1/P_{cr}$, (b) GFR, (c) the rate of creatinine excretion, (d) fractional excretion of water, and (e) absolute and fractional rates of Na excretion.

9. A subject with stable chronic renal failure is given a drug to control gastric acid production (cimetidine). The following values were obtained immediately before and 4 days after the drug was started. (a) Calculate the creatinine and urea clearances for the two sets of values. (b) Calculate the excretion rates for creatinine and urea for the two sets of values. (c) How can you explain the different effect of the drug on the clearances of creatinine and urea?

	Baseline	After Cimetidine
Plasma creatinine	2.8 mg/dl	3.4
Urine creatinine	41.2 mg/dl	38.2
Plasma urea nitrogen	32.0 mg/dl	32.2
Urine urea nitrogen	316 mg/dl	296
Urine volume (24 hour)	2040 ml/day	2160

10. The clearance of substance A is less than that simultaneously determined for inulin. Give three possible explanations.

11. In a normal subject, the urea clearance was found to be 60% of the inulin clearance, which was 120 ml/min. The plasma concentration of urea was 0.12 mg/ml. How much urea was reabsorbed by the tubules?

12. If there are 0.004 gm/100 ml of protein in the glomerular filtrate and no protein is reabsorbed, what would be the amount of protein excreted per day?

13. In a normal man with a urine flow of 0.5 ml per minute, a substance present in the plasma in a concentration of 0.5 mg/100 ml appears in the urine in a concentration of 280 mg/100 ml. How is this substance being excreted by the kidney?

ANSWERS TO PROBLEMS

1. GFR = C_{in} = $U_{in} \dot{V}/P_{in}$ Period 1: 106 ml/min   Period 7: 109 ml/min

2. a. RPF = C_{PAH} in the first three periods. In the later periods, Tm_{PAH} is approached and RPF $\neq$ C_{PAH}.

RPF = 620, 611, and 625 ml/min in first three periods.
Average: 619 ml/min.

b. RBF = RPF/(1 − Hct) = 1088, 1053, and 1078 ml/min in first three periods.   Average = 1073 ml/min.

c. Tm_G can be calculated when the transport system is saturated. Saturation can be inferred when P_G increases in consecutive periods but T_G does not. That condition exists in periods 6 and 7.

$$T_G = P_G GFR - U_G \dot{V} = 370 \text{ and } 369 \text{ mg/min.}$$

d. The same type of criteria can be applied to the determination of Tm_{PAH}.

$$T_{PAH} = U_{PAH}\dot{V} - P_{PAH}GFR = 81.6, 80.4, \text{ and } 82.3 \text{ mg/min in}$$
periods 5, 6, and 7.   Average: 81.4 mg/min.

3. As P_G increases, the amount filtered increases ($P_G \cdot$ GFR). However, at a certain point, the transport system becomes saturated and T_G increases no further. A greater fraction of the filtered load is excreted as P_G increases, and thus the volume of plasma cleared of glucose increases. Other substances that are reabsorbed will show the same pattern. As P_{PAH} increases, the amount presented for secretion (P_{PAH}RPF) increases. However, after the secretory system is saturated, a constant amount is secreted as the amount presented for secretion increases, thus a smaller fraction of the plasma flow is cleared of PAH. Other substances that are secreted would follow the same pattern.

4. a. $C_{cr} = U_{cr}\dot{V}/P_{cr} = 118$ ml/min

   b. Fractional water excretion = $\dot{V}/$GFR or $\dot{V}/C_{cr}$ = .0075 or 0.75%.

   $$\text{Also } \dot{V}/C_{cr} = \frac{\dot{V}}{U_{cr}\dot{V}/P_{cr}} = \frac{1}{U_{cr}/P_{cr}} = \frac{P_{cr}}{U_{cr}} = .0075$$

   c. Fractional water reabsorption = (GFR − $\dot{V}$)/GFR = 1 − $\dot{V}$/GFR
   = 1 − $\dot{V}/C_{cr}$ = 1 − P_{cr}/U_{cr} = .9925 or 99.25%.

5. $FE_{H_2O} = P_{cr}/U_{cr}$, $FR_{H_2O} = 1 - P_{cr}/U_{cr}$

	FE_{H_2O}	FR_{H_2O}
a.	50.0%	50.0%
b.	21.1	78.9
c.	2.9	97.1
d.	0.93	99.07
e.	0.24	99.76

6. a. C_{cr} = 75.5 ml/min

   b. Rate of filtration of Na = P_{Na} × GFR = 10570 μEq/min, 10.57 mEq/min and 15.22 Eq/day.

   c. Rate of Na excretion = $U_{Na} \dot{V}$ = 54.4 μEq/min, .0544 mEq/min or 78.3 mEq/day

   d. FE_{Na} = $(U/P)_{Na}/(U/P)_{cr}$ = 0.51% FR_{Na} = 100 − 0.51 = 99.49%

   e. FE_{urate} = $(U/P)_{urate}/(U/P)_{cr}$ = 10.1%

7. a. C_{cr} = $U_{cr} \dot{V}/P_{cr}$ = 7.9 ml/min

   b. FE_{Na} = 4.7%; FE_K = 148%; FE_{PO_4} = 38.2%

   c. Potassium secretion

8. a. $1/P_{cr}$ in patient 6 = 1.11; in patient 7 = 0.12.

   b. GFR in patient 6 = 75.5 ml/min; in patient 7 = 7.9 ml/min.

   c. Rate of creatinine excretion = $U_{cr} \dot{V}$

   Patient 6: 979 mg/day; patient 7: 972 mg/day.

   The values of $1/P_{cr}$ indicate that glomerular function is greatly reduced in patient 7. This is verified by calculation of GFR. The values for patient 6 fall in the normal range. Despite the fall in creatinine clearance, patient 7 is still able to excrete creatinine at the same rate as patient 6. Creatinine excretion is primarily dependent on the rate at which it is filtered. When GFR falls, the rate of excretion falls momentarily, causing the plasma concentration to rise (the rate of creatinine production is assumed to remain constant). This causes the rate of creatinine filtration ($P_{cr} \cdot$ GFR) to return to its former level, and the rate of excretion then also returns to its previous level. Thus in patient 7, the increase in P_{cr} counterbalances the fall in GFR, so that the rate of excretion remains equal to the production rate.

   d. Fractional water excretion = P_{cr}/U_{cr}.

   Patient 6: 0.8%; patient 7: 15.7%.

   e. Absolute Na excretion rate = $U_{Na} \dot{V}$

   Patient 6: 78.3 mEq/day; patient 7: 72 mEq/day.

   Fractional Na excretion = $(U/P)_{Na}/(U/P)_{cr}$.

   Patient 6: 0.51%; patient 7: 4.7%.

   The decreased GFR in patient 7 tends to increase the retention of salt and water. This triggers several factors that reduce salt and water reabsorption by the tubules (see Chapter 9). Thus, patient 7 can excrete as much water and almost as much Na as patient 6.

9.		Baseline	After Cimetidine
a.	C_{cr}	20.8 ml/min	16.9 ml/min
	C_U	14.0	13.8
b.	Creatinine excretion	840 mg/day	825 mg/day
	Urea excretion	6446	6394

    c. The drug did not alter the rate of excretion of creatinine or urea, nor the clearance of urea. The reduced clearance of creatinine may be explained by an effect of the drug that blocks creatinine secretion into the renal tubule.

10. a. Reabsorption

    b. Not filtered because it is too large.

    c. Not filtered because it is bound to plasma protein.

11. $C_U/C_{in} = (U/P)_U/(U/P)_{in} = 0.6$. Thus $FE_U = 60\%$ and $FR_U = 40\%$. The amount filtered $= P_U C_{in}$, so the amount reabsorbed $= 0.4\ P_U C_{in} = 5.76$ mg/min.

12. Assume normal GFR of 180 L/day. Answer: 7.2 gm/day.

13. $C_X = 280$ ml/min. This is more than twice the normal clearance rate of inulin, indicating that plasma must be cleared of the substance by tubular secretion in addition to filtration.

BIBLIOGRAPHY

Clearance Methods:

Brenner, B. M., Ichikawa, I., and Deen, W. M.: Glomerular Filtration. *In* The Kidney, 2nd ed. Vol. 1. Edited by B. M. Brenner, and F. C., Rector, Jr. Philadelphia, W. B. Saunders Co., 1981.

Pitts, R. F.: Physiology of the Kidney and Body Fluids. 3rd ed. Chicago, Year Book Medical Publishers, Inc., 1974.

Smith, H.W.: Principles of Renal Physiology. New York, Oxford University Press, 1956.

Wesson, L. G., Jr.: Physiology of Human Kidney. New York, Grune and Stratton, 1969.

Research Methods:

Burg, M., Grantham, J., Abramow, M., and Orloff, J.: Preparation and study of fragments of single rabbit nephrons. Am. J. Physiol., *210*:1293, 1966.

Chonko, A. M., Irish, J. M. III, and Welling, D. J.: Microperfusion of Isolated Tubules. *In* Methods in Pharmacology Vol. 4B. Edited by M. Martinez-Maldonado. New York, Plenum Publishing Corp., 1978.

Malvin, R. L., Wilde, W. S., and Sullivan, L. P.: Localization of nephron transport by stop flow analysis. Am. J. Physiol., *194*:135, 1958.

See the following chapters from: Orloff, J., and Berliner, R. W.: Renal Physiology Sec. 8 of Handbook of Physiology. Washington, D. C. Am. Physiol. Soc., 1973.

    Chapter 5: Malvin, R. L., and Wilde, W. S.: Stop-Flow Technique.

    Chapter 6: Gottschalk, C. W., and Lassiter, W. E.: Micropuncture Methodology.

    Chapter 7: Burg, M. B., and Orloff, J.: Perfusion of Isolated Renal Tubules.

See also the following Chapters from: Passow, H., and Stämpfli, R. (Eds): Laboratory Methods in Membrane Biophysics. New York, Springer-Verlag, 1969.

Clarkson, T. W., and Lindemann, B.: Experiments on Na Transport of Frog Skin Epithelium.

Ullrich, K. J., Frömter, E., and Baumann, K.: Micropuncture and Microanalysis in Kidney Physiology.

CHAPTER *4*

Blood Flow and Filtration

The kidney is a highly vascular organ that normally provides little resistance to blood flow through it. Consequently, the two kidneys, which together comprise less than 0.5% of body weight, usually receive 20 to 25% of the cardiac output, about 1000 to 1200 ml/min. Of the 600 to 700 ml of plasma contained in that blood, about 120 ml are filtered per minute from the glomerular capillaries into the tubules. All but 1 to 2 ml of that is subsequently reabsorbed and returned to the circulation via the peritubular capillaries. Control of the rate of blood flow is complex and involves extrinsic neural and humoral factors and an intrinsic control system. Control of the blood flow rate is also intimately tied to control of the glomerular filtration rate. This chapter describes the relevant anatomy, the filtering process, the mechanisms controlling blood flow and filtration, and their regulation. Later chapters will describe the multiple processes involved in the reabsorption and return of fluid and solute to the circulation.

PRESSURE GRADIENTS AND CONTROL POINTS

Figure 4-1 illustrates the changes that occur in the hydrostatic pressure of blood as it flows from the renal artery through the arterioles and capillary beds into the renal vein. The largest falls in pressure occur in the afferent and efferent arterioles. These are the sites of greatest resistance to flow, and therefore, the major sites of control of blood flow. The unique positioning of the glomerular capillary bed between these two major resistance sites permits the maintenance of a relatively high hydrostatic pressure in that bed and also provides a mechanism for close control of the pressure and flow. By controlling pressure and flow the arterioles also control the rate of filtration through the capillary wall. Normally, 18 to 20% of the plasma flow is filtered into the tubules. The glomerular capillary membrane is relatively impermeable to protein, so the loss of the protein-free filtrate raises the colloid osmotic or oncotic

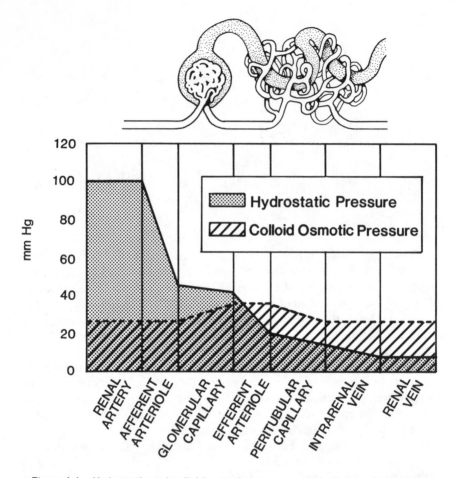

Figure 4-1. Hydrostatic and colloid osmotic pressures within the renal vasculature.

pressure (π_b) of the remaining 80 to 82% of the plasma, as illustrated in Figure 4-1.

In the peritubular capillary bed, the hydrostatic pressure is low because of the high resistance sites located upstream. In addition, the colloid osmotic pressure of the plasma flowing into the peritubular capillaries is high because of the filtration of protein-free fluid that occurs in the glomerular capillaries. The balance between the two pressures causes an osmotic flow of fluid, which has been reabsorbed from the tubules, back into the bloodstream. The addition of that fluid causes π_b to decline toward the initial level existing in plasma entering the renal artery.

THE JUXTAGLOMERULAR APPARATUS

Each nephron forms a loop so that the beginning of the distal tubule comes into close contact with the glomerulus and the afferent and efferent arterioles, the two major sites of control of blood flow and filtration rate (Fig. 2-2). This conjunction of the arterioles, glomerulus, and distal tubule of one vascular-tubular unit is called the juxtaglomerular apparatus. The details of its structure are presented in Figure 4-2.

Specialized cells appear in the wall of the tubule and the arterioles at the site of their contact. Large columnar cells, called macula densa cells, in the wall of the distal tubule are in contact with the granular cells in the wall of the afferent and efferent arterioles. Another group of cells appears between the two arterioles. These have been called variously the lacis, the polkissen (polar cushion), and the extraglomerular mesangium. Granular cells may also occasionally appear in the lacis. In addition to their contact with the granular cells, the macula densa cells also interdigitate with cells in the lacis. These macula densa cells may provide information on the volume or composition of the tubular con-

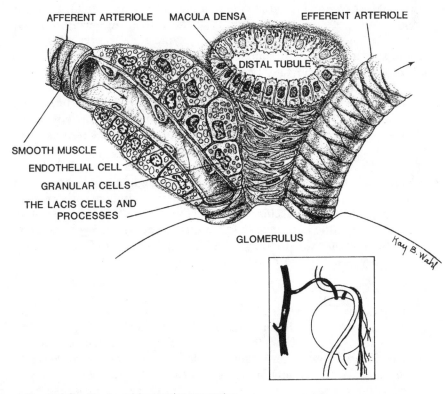

Figure 4-2. The juxtaglomerular apparatus.

tents to the juxtaglomerular apparatus. As the inset in Figure 4-2 shows, the area of contact between the distal tubule and efferent arteriole is much greater than that between the tubule and the afferent arteriole. The physiologic significance of this is not known.

The body can effect changes in the degree of constriction of the afferent and efferent arterioles through humoral factors arriving via the blood stream, through stimuli carried by the nerves innervating the juxtaglomerular apparatus, and through stimuli carried by the tubular fluid and transmitted by the macula densa. These changes in arteriolar resistance affect RBF, glomerular capillary pressure, and GFR. In turn, the juxtaglomerular apparatus can exert a profound influence on blood pressure, blood flow, and extracellular fluid volume throughout the body by altering the rate of filtration and by releasing renin into the circulation.

The enzyme renin splits a decapeptide from the alpha-2-globulin fraction of plasma protein. This decapeptide is angiotensin I, which loses two amino acids in the presence of a converting enzyme to become the octapeptide angiotensin II. This is the active form which acts as a vasoconstrictor and causes the secretion of aldosterone by the adrenal cortex. Most of the angiotensin I is converted to angiotensin II by the lungs, which contain large amounts of the converting enzyme. However, small amounts of the converting enzyme are also present in renal tissue and in plasma. In some tissues, such as the adrenal cortex, an additional amino acid may be split off to form angiotensin III, which may exert its effect only at the site of its formation.

The stimuli for renin release from the granular cells, like the stimuli for changes in constriction of the arterioles, may be carried by the bloodstream, by the nerves, and by the tubular fluid. The renin system plays a role in the maintenance of arterial pressure both by the vasoconstrictor effect of angiotensin II and by its effect on extracellular fluid volume through its influence on aldosterone. Angiotensin II, because of its potent vasoconstrictor action, probably is the principal pathophysiologic mediator of renovascular hypertension. The influence of angiotensin on ECF volume is discussed in Chapter Nine. It has been hypothesized that angiotensin also plays a role in regulation of renal blood flow. This theory is described below.

THE GLOMERULUS

The glomerulus consists of a group or tuft of specialized capillaries situated between an afferent and an efferent arteriole (Fig. 4-3). The capillary loops are held together by mesangial cells, which act much in the same way as the larger mesentery of the intestines. These cells also serve other functions such as phagocytosis of macromolecular aggregates. The mesangium also contains contractile elements whose function is not known. The capillary tuft projects into Bowman's capsule,

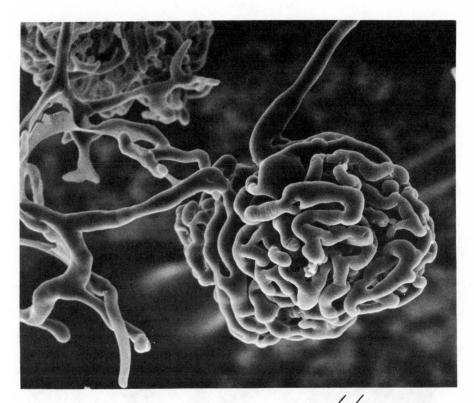

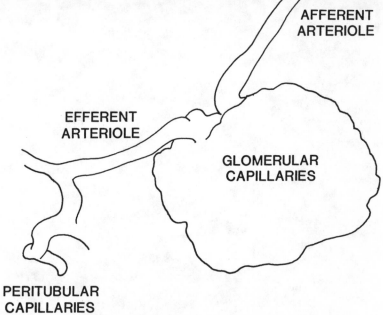

AFFERENT
ARTERIOLE

EFFERENT
ARTERIOLE

GLOMERULAR
CAPILLARIES

PERITUBULAR
CAPILLARIES

Figure 4-3.   (A) Scanning electron micrograph of a cast of a glomerular capillary tuft.
(Courtesy of Dr. Andrew Evan.) (B) identification of structures that appear in A.

which is a hollow sphere lined by a single layer of epithelial cells. A complex interdigitating network of epithelial cells lines the outer surface of glomerular capillaries, as illustrated in Figures 4-4 and 4-5. These epithelial cells, called podocytes, send out foot processes which interdigitate with foot processes from neighboring cells. The endothelium lining the inner surface of the capillaries is penetrated by openings or fenestrations of about 600 to 1000 Å in diameter (Fig. 4-5). These fenestrations take up a large portion of the surface area.

Fluid leaving the capillary and entering Bowman's capsule must pass through the three layers that comprise the capillary wall: the capillary endothelium, a basement membrane, and the epithelial cell layer. Figure 4-6 is a transmission electron micrograph of a cross section of the capillary wall and Figure 4-7 is a drawing that emphasizes the major features of this structure. The fenestrations in the capillary endothelium may be covered by a thin diaphragm, but in any case, they are easily penetrated by compounds of large molecular weight but not by the cellular elements of the blood. The basement membrane is composed of a dense layer, the lamina densa, sandwiched between two less dense layers, the lamina rara interna and externa. The foot processes of the

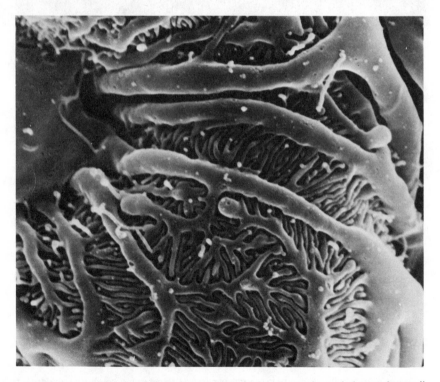

Figure 4-4. Scanning electron micrograph of the outer surface of glomerular capillaries. (Courtesy of Dr. Andrew Evan.)

MESANGIUM ⌐

ENDOTHELIUM ⌐

FOOT PROCESS ⌐   PODOCYTE ⌐

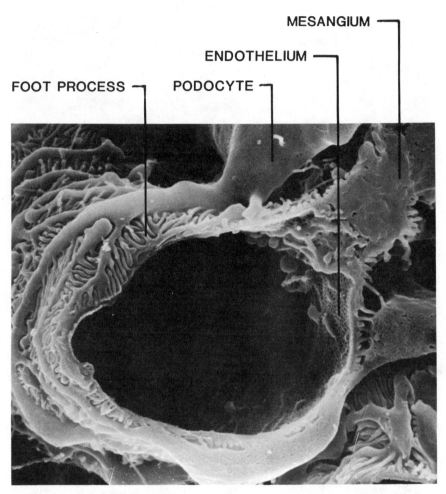

Figure 4-5.   Scanning electron micrograph of the outer and inner surface of a glomerular capillary. (Courtesy of Dr. Andrew Evan.)

epithelial cell layer are separated by channels or slits that may be approximately 240 Å in width and 3000 to 5000 Å in height. Neighboring foot processes are connected at their base by a slit membrane, which is also the outer limiting membrane of the basement membrane. Glycoproteins coat both the endothelial and the epithelial cell membranes, cover the endothelial fenestrations, and fill the slits or channels between the foot processes. In addition, the basement membrane consists to a large extent of glycoproteins and collagen. The glycoproteins contain sialic acid, which confers a strong negative charge to the cell coating and the basement membrane. The collagen probably gives structural strength to the basement membrane.

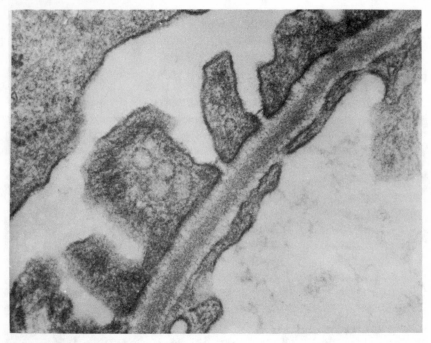

Figure 4-6. Transmission electron micrograph of the glomerular capillary wall. (Courtesy of Dr. Francis Cuppage.)

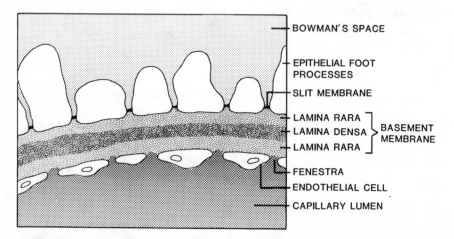

Figure 4-7. The structure of the glomerular capillary wall, the filtering pathway.

The filtration pathway through the fenestration, across the basement membrane and the slit membrane, and through the slits provides little hindrance to the passage of solutes with a molecular weight up to 5000 (molecular radius, 14 Å). Above that point, the ability of macromolecules to penetrate the barrier is a function of their shape, size, and ionic charge. Elongated, flexible molecules can penetrate the glomerular membrane more easily than globular molecules. Neutral macromolecules of dextran, up to 20 Å in radius, are not hindered in crossing the glomerular membrane, but the penetrating ability of larger molecules decreases rapidly with size. Negatively charged macromolecules are evidently repelled by the fixed negative charges present in the basement membrane and the glycoprotein cell coating. Conversely, positively charged molecules can penetrate the glomerular membrane more easily than neutral molecules of the same size. Table 4-1 compares the fractional clearance of the plasma protein albumin with dextran molecules of the same molecular radius. Dextran sulfate is negatively charged and its fractional clearance is much less than that of neutral dextran. Albumin is a polyanion at plasma pH, and its low fractional clearance is due not only to its size but also to its negative charges. The shape of the albumin molecule may also reduce its fractional clearance somewhat.

TABLE 4.1 FRACTIONAL CLEARANCE OF ALBUMIN AND SELECTED DEXTRAN MOLECULES

Macromolecule (M)	Molecular Radius (Å)	Fractional Clearance $(U/P)_m / (U/P)_{in}$
Normal values		
Albumin	36	< 0.001
Neutral dextran	36	0.19
Dextran sulfate	36	0.015
Experimental glomerular nephritis		
Neutral dextran	36	0.14
Dextran sulfate	36	0.24

Disease processes affect the glomerulus in several different ways. In glomerulonephritis, immune complexes are deposited in the glomerular capillary walls. The deposits interact with complement in the blood and then attract leukocytes, which in turn, release proteolytic enzymes that produce minute holes in the capillaries. Erythrocytes and plasma can then leak into Bowman's space and, eventually, into the final urine. Some diseases evidently change the net charge on the glycoproteins coating the glomerular capillaries, allowing proteins like albumin to cross the glomerular barrier more easily and leak into the urine. In these states, one sees excessive protein but not erythrocytes in the urine.

Table 4-1 illustrates how one form of glomerulonephritis, induced experimentally in rats, reduces to some extent the ability of neutral dextran with the same molecular radius as serum albumin to penetrate the glomerular capillary. This suggests that the disease may cause the loss of capillary surface area through which protein can enter Bowman's space. In contrast, the fractional clearance of negatively charged dextran sulfate of the same radius is greatly increased. Evidently, the disease process has caused the loss of fixed negative charges from the membrane, enabling negatively charged macromolecules like albumin to penetrate the membrane more easily and appear in the urine to a much greater extent.

COMPOSITION OF THE FILTRATE

The fluid crossing the glomerular membrane and entering the capsular space is an ultrafiltrate of plasma, containing all the substances that exist in plasma except the proteins. The concentrations of these substances in the filtrate are the same as in plasma except for some minor variations in electrolyte concentrations due to the Donnan forces that result from the protein concentration differences between plasma and the ultrafiltrate. A variety of substances, including many foreign compounds, are bound to the plasma proteins to a varying extent. The bound fraction is not filtered but the free portion is. These exceptions are minor, and it is emphasized that the composition of the ultrafiltrate is almost identical to the composition of plasma except for the proteins.

FORCES INVOLVED IN GLOMERULAR FILTRATION

The major force inducing filtration of water and solutes across the glomerular membrane is the intracapillary hydrostatic pressure, which ultimately results from the contraction of the heart. This pressure is determined by the aortic pressure and the resistances to blood flow provided by the afferent and efferent arterioles (Fig. 4-1). This glomerular capillary hydrostatic pressure (P_{gc}) is opposed by two forces: the capsular or tubular hydrostatic pressure (P_t) and the effective osmotic pressure of the blood in the capillary (π_b) (Fig. 4-8). As has already been stated, the filtering surface is permeable to all substances in plasma except protein, so only the protein exerts an effective osmotic pressure; this is called the colloid osmotic or oncotic pressure. Since the capsular fluid contains only traces of protein, it exerts no effective osmotic pressure on the glomerular membrane. Thus, at any point along the glomerular capillary bed, the net filtration pressure (P_f) can be expressed as

$$P_f = P_{gc} - P_t - \pi_b$$

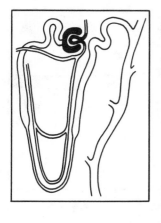 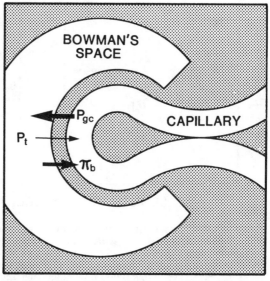

$$P_f = P_{gc} - (P_t + \pi_b)$$

Figure 4-8. The pressures involved in glomerular filtration. P_{gc} = capillary hydrostatic pressure. P_t = tubular or Bowman's space hydrostatic pressure. π_b = colloid osmotic pressure of plasma. P_f = net filtration pressure.

It is useful to express the hydrostatic pressure gradient across the capillary wall ($P_{gc} - P_t$) as $\triangle P$; thus

$$P_f = \triangle P - \pi_b$$

Figure 4-9A illustrates the changes that occur in $\triangle P$ and π_b along the length of the glomerular capillary bed. Because of the high resistance to flow downstream in the efferent arteriole, P_{gc} and thus $\triangle P$ drop only slightly along the bed. π_b rises as plasma traverses the capillaries because the loss of protein-free fluid from the plasma by filtration raises the protein concentration of the remaining plasma. As a result, the net filtration pressure (P_f), represented by the shaded area in the graph, decreases along the length of the bed.

The magnitude of the rise in π_b is proportional to the fraction of the total plasma flow that is filtered (GFR/RPF). Figure 4-9B illustrates what happens to π_b, and therefore to P_f, when the plasma flow rate rises. A smaller fraction of that larger flow rate is filtered and thus the increase in π_b is not as great. This results in a greater P_f at each point along the length of the capillary bed. Theoretically, this should cause a greater rate of filtration.

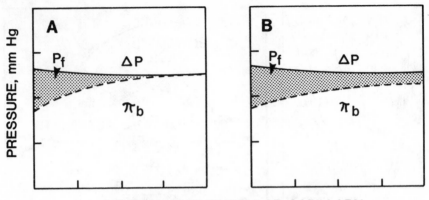

Figure 4-9. Pressure gradients along the length of the glomerular capillaries. $\Delta P = P_{gc} - P_t =$ the hydrostatic pressure gradient across the capillary wall and is indicated by the solid line. π_b is the colloid osmotic pressure of the plasma and is represented by the dashed curve. $P_f = \Delta P - \pi_b =$ net filtration pressure and is indicated by the shaded areas. (A) Pressures at low blood flow rates. This figure also represents the pressure curves that have been measured in the rat and monkey under control conditions. (B) Pressures at high blood flow rates. This figure also represents the pressure gradients that probably exist normally in the dog.

Figure 4-9 also serves to illustrate one of the current quandaries in renal physiology. Figure 4-9A shows the type of curves that have been obtained in experiments on the rat and on one species of monkey. At the distal end of the capillary, π_b has risen to equal ΔP, so P_f is zero. There is then a fraction of the total capillary bed across which no filtration is occurring. This "reserve" fraction of the filtering surface could be utilized if ΔP were increased or if the plasma flow rate were increased so that the increase in the opposing pressure (π_b) were less, as in Figure 4-9B. The normal situation that probably exists in the dog is illustrated in Figure 4-9B. Indirect measurements indicate that there is a net P_f at the distal end of the glomerular capillaries, and the entire filtering surface is evidently utilized normally. A rise in ΔP increases the filtration rate, but not quite to the same extent as in the rat (Fig. 4-9A), because the area utilized for filtration does not increase. A rise in plasma flow has even less of an effect, not only because the filtering area does not change but also because further flattening of the π_b curve does not increase P_f to the same extent as in the rat. Table 4-2 lists the values for the relevant pressures in the rat, dog, and monkey. Anesthesia, surgical trauma, blood loss, and variable arterial plasma protein concentrations complicate the interpretation of these experimental data. No pertinent data are available for man.

The rate of filtration of fluid by the glomerular capillaries depends not only upon the pressures involved, but also upon the physical characteristics of the filtering surface, that is, the hydraulic or water permeability (L_p) of the glomerular membrane and its surface area, A. These two values are difficult to determine separately but their product, the filtration coefficient (k_f) can be calculated from measurements of GFR and $\overline{P}_f$. Values for these factors are listed in Table 4-2. The hydraulic permeability of the glomerular capillaries is 10 to 100 times greater than that of capillaries elsewhere in the body.

TABLE 4-2   FACTORS INVOLVED IN GLOMERULAR FILTRATION

	RAT	DOG	MONKEY
P_{gc}, mm Hg	45	55–60	49
P_t , mm Hg	12	20	13
π_b , mm Hg, afferent end	20	21	24
π_b , mm Hg, efferent end	35	33	37
P_f , mm Hg, afferent end	15	15–20	12
P_f , mm Hg, efferent end	0	10	0
A , surface area for filtration mm² per glomerulus	0.2	0.4	—
L_p , hydraulic permeability, $nl \cdot sec^{-1} \cdot mm\ Hg^{-1} \cdot cm^{-2}$	29	16–18	
L_pA = k_f, filtration coefficient $nl \cdot min^{-1} \cdot mm\ Hg^{-1}$	3.5	4.2	
GFR = $k_f\overline{P}_f$, $nl \cdot min^{-1}$ per glomerulus	28	55	17

FACTORS AFFECTING GFR

The glomerular filtration rate can be altered by changes in any one of the pressures involved or by changes in k_f. Usually, changes in more than just one factor are involved in any alteration of GFR. P_{gc} can be altered by changes in arterial pressure and by changes in afferent and efferent arteriolar resistance. Dilution or loss of plasma proteins decreases π_b. Changes in plasma flow rate affect the rate of increase in π_b within glomerular capillaries as described earlier and in Figure 4-9. Ureteral, calyceal, or tubular obstruction increases P_t and reduces GFR. Alterations in k_f may occur physiologically and in glomerular disease. These alterations may be the result of changes in hydraulic permeability or in glomerular capillary surface area or both.

The two major sites of control of GFR are the afferent and efferent arterioles. Changes in the degree of constriction of smooth muscle in the wall of one or both arterioles alter the resistance to flow and thereby change the pressure and flow rate in the glomerular capillaries. Constriction of the afferent arteriole causes the pressure downstream to fall and this tends to lower GFR. Since the plasma flow rate also decreases, the rate of rise in π_b is increased, and this too tends to reduce GFR. Constriction of the efferent arteriole causes P_{gc} upstream to rise and this tends to increase GFR. However, the increase in resistance reduces the RPF and the resulting effect on π_b tends to reduce GFR. Thus, the net effect of efferent arteriolar constriction alone on GFR is difficult to predict. Resolution of this question depends in part on an answer to the question: to what extent does π_b increase during filtration?

It is apparent that the major sites for control of GFR are also the sites for control of RPF. A variety of neural and humoral factors can act upon the afferent and efferent arterioles to change their degree of constriction so that resistance to flow and glomerular capillary pressures are altered. These factors may also alter k_f. In addition, hydrostatic and oncotic pressures downstream in the peritubular capillary bed are affected.

FACTORS AFFECTING THE ARTERIOLES

The resistance to flow provided by the afferent and efferent arterioles is determined primarily by the contractile state of the arteriolar smooth muscle. A resting tone is maintained by intrinsic myogenic activity. This tone can be abolished and RBF can be increased 50 to 100% by smooth muscle relaxants such as papaverine or acetylcholine. The level of this tone is low compared to other organs, and as pointed out above, the blood flow per gram of tissue is high. Another consequence of this relatively low tone is that the *fractional* capacity to increase flow by vasodilation is lower than in other organs. However, in *absolute* terms, a 50 to 100% increase in a flow that is already equivalent to 20% of the cardiac output is large.

A consequence of the low resistance to flow is that, unlike the situation in other capillary beds, the individual capillaries in the glomerular and peritubular beds are evidently always open and there is always some degree of flow through them. In other words, there is no intermittent flow in single capillaries.

The factors that act on the juxtaglomerular apparatus to alter the resting tone of the arteriolar smooth muscle arise both from outside and inside the kidney. Sympathetic vasoconstrictor fibers, arising primarily from the celiac ganglia, innervate both arterioles within the juxtaglomerular apparatus. They also reach the initial segments of the vasa recta which contain smooth muscle cells. There are no sympathetic vasodilator fibers. Cholinergic, parasympathetic fibers, arising apparently from ganglia in the hilus or in the renal parenchyma, also innervate both arterioles. Although it might be expected that these fibers would cause vasodilation, no convincing evidence of this has yet been found.

A variety of humoral factors can be carried to the arterioles. Both α and β receptors for catecholamines are present. The α receptors greatly outnumber β receptors however, and all dose levels of either epinephrine or norepinephrine cause only vasoconstriction. Acetylcholine causes vasodilation. Pyrogens produced as a result of infection by bacteria, viruses, molds, or yeast also cause vasodilation.

The kidney also produces a number of vasoactive substances that can influence arteriolar constriction. The release of renin results in the formation of angiotensin I, which is converted to the active form angiotensin II by the lungs. This active form is returned to the kidney via the circulation and can cause vasoconstriction. In addition, small amounts of angiotensin II can be formed within the kidneys and have the same effect. The drug saralasin, which is a closely related octapeptide, blocks the effects of angiotensin II. Captopril is a drug that blocks conversion of angiotensin I to angiotensin II.

A second hormonal system is interrelated with the renin–angiotensin system. The enzyme kallikrein is formed and stored in the cortex. Upon release, it causes the liberation of a peptide, bradykinin, from plasma globulins. Bradykinin is a vasodilator. The enzyme that converts angiotensin I to angiotensin II also degrades bradykinin. In other words, the converting enzyme activates a vasoconstrictor and deactivates a vasodilator. Most of the renin released by the kidney leaves via the renal vein, but kallikrein exits in the urine.

Prostaglandin E_2, a vasodilator, is produced in the cortical and medullary areas of the kidney. Prostaglandin produced in the medullary area may be carried to the cortex and the juxtaglomerular apparatus by the tubular fluid. The substrate for prostaglandin synthesis is arachidonic acid. The synthesis can be blocked by indomethacin and meclofenamate. There is evidence of close interrelationships between prostaglandin on the one hand and the renin–angiotensin and kallikrein–bradykinin systems on the other. These relationships are not yet fully delineated.

Dopamine is present in high concentrations in the cortex, and specific receptors for it may exist there. The physiologic significance of this finding is not known. Pharmacologically, small doses of dopamine cause vasodilation, and this effect is considered to be mediated by the specific receptors. High doses cause vasoconstriction, which is mediated by α receptors.

In many tissues, local changes in the partial pressure of oxygen and carbon dioxide and the accumulation of other metabolites alter the degree of vasoconstriction. This probably does not occur in the kidney. It receives far more oxygen than it requires and the arteriovenous oxygen difference is only 1 to 2 vol %. In contrast to other tissues, oxygen consumption varies with blood flow and the arteriovenous oxygen difference does not change when blood flow does. The explanation for this is based on the fact that the reabsorption of Na accounts for over half of the oxygen consumed by the kidney. To the extent that the magnitude of the blood flow determines the filtration rate and the amount of sodium presented for reabsorption, it also determines the amount of work to be done and the amount of oxygen to be consumed. This also explains the observation that there is little renal hyperemia following ischemia. Unlike the situation in muscle, for example, reduction in blood flow decreases the amount of work to be done and little oxygen debt is accumulated.

An additional factor, which is purely physical, may play a role in regulation of RBF and GFR. It has been proposed that the arteriolar smooth muscle reacts directly to changes in blood pressure. All smooth muscle responds to stretch by increasing the active tension generated by the contractile fibers. The response of the arteriolar smooth muscle to a rise in pressure in the lumen may be to contract and reduce the diameter of the lumen, thereby increasing resistance to flow.

REGULATION OF RBF AND GFR.

Intrinsic or Autoregulation

In attempting to study the processes by which RBF and GFR are regulated, experiments were performed to determine the response of the kidney to variations in arterial pressure when the effects of extrinsic controlling factors are eliminated. In these experiments, the renal nerves were severed and the effects of sympathomimetic amines were eliminated either by the use of blocking agents or by removing the adrenal medulla. Renal arterial pressure was either elevated by stimulation of the sympathetic nervous system or reduced by partially clamping the dorsal aorta above the origin of the renal artery. The results obtained in experiments of this type are illustrated in Figure 4-10. Over the renal arterial pressure range of about 80 to 180 mm Hg, both RBF and GFR are maintained relatively constant. Thus, in the absence of extrinsic influences, intrinsic mechanisms enable the kidney to autoregulate GFR and RBF. The fact that GFR is maintained constant indicates that P_{gc}, as well as glomerular plasma flow, is kept constant. It is apparent then, that resistance upstream from the glomerular capillaries in the afferent arteriole must change as renal artery pressure changes. Efferent arteriolar resistance may change also, but it is obvious that the major change occurs in the afferent arteriole.

This autoregulatory response of the kidney has been clearly and amply documented, but the mechanism or mechanisms responsible still elude our understanding. It is clear that changes in constriction of the arterioles are involved, since papaverine, an arteriolar muscle relaxant, abolishes autoregulation. However, we do not know what signal is perceived nor how it ultimately results in a change in arteriolar tone. It is apparent that the signal is not the partial pressure of oxygen or carbon dioxide in the tissue nor the accumulation of metabolites. One major

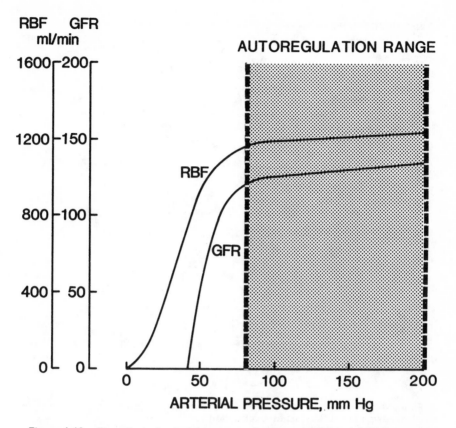

Figure 4-10. The effect of arterial pressure changes on RBF and GFR. In the absence of extrinsic regulation, the kidney itself maintains both GFR and RBF relatively constant over the range of pressure from 80 to 200 mm Hg.

theory suggests that a change in pressure or tension in the arterioles is the primary stimulus and the response is the direct smooth muscle reaction to stretch. However, there are theoretical objections to the idea that the arterioles can respond directly to changes in tension in such a manner that flow through the arteriole can be kept constant. It may be that smooth muscle contractility is mediated by an agent that is released in response to a change in pressure.

Recently, it has been argued that the kidney regulates GFR primarily and that RBF regulation is a secondary consequence of controlling GFR. This theory is based on the results of the following type of experiment (Fig. 4-11). Utilizing the micropuncture technique, a pipette is inserted into an early segment of the proximal tubule and a column of oil is injected to block flow downstream. Fluid arriving at the puncture site is collected, and with the use of inulin, the filtration rate for that single

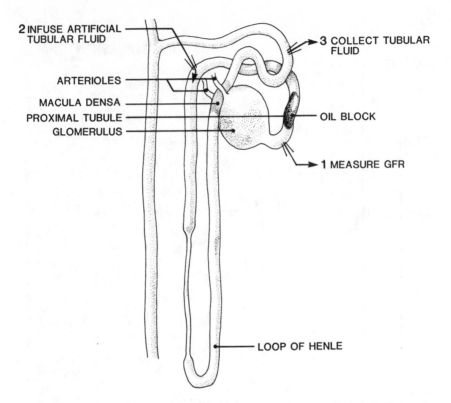

Figure 4-11. Illustration of an experiment designed to test the tubuloglomerular feedback hypothesis. See text for explanation.

glomerulus is measured (Fig. 4-11—1). Another pipette is inserted into a later segment of that proximal tubule, distal to the oil block, and artificial tubular fluid is perfused at varying rates (Fig. 4-11—2). A third pipette can be inserted into the distal tubule just beyond the macula densa to measure the rate and composition of the perfusate arriving at that point (Fig. 4-11—3). The results obtained from this type of experiment indicate that the filtration rate in that nephron falls as the rate of perfusion of the segment of the tubule containing the macula densa cells increases. This leads to the conclusion that an increase in the single nephron glomerular filtration rate (SN GFR) in an intact nephron causes an increase in the tubular fluid flow rate past the macula densa cells, which somehow results in a fall in P_{gc} so that SN GFR returns to its control level (Fig. 4-12). Thus, it is proposed that each nephron regulates its own filtration rate. This mechanism has been given the awkward name "tubulo-glomerular feedback mechanism." It is suggested that as a consequence of each nephron regulating its filtration rate by this device, whole-kidney GFR, and secondarily RBF, are autoregulated.

The receptor for this mechanism is presumed to be the macula densa cells. The exact signal to which they respond is not known. It is in some way related to the tubular fluid flow rate and may possibly be the rate of delivery of salt to that tubular site. How that signal is transduced to a stimulus that alters arteriolar constriction is not known. It has been repeatedly suggested that an increase in salt delivery to the macula densa increases renin release by the juxtaglomerular apparatus and formation of angiotensin at that site. The angiotensin then causes arteriolar constriction. There is one major stumbling block to this proposal. It requires that renin release increase in response to a rise in GFR. However, it is in precisely the opposite situation, when GFR and RBF fall, that increased renin levels are found in renal venous blood. It is possible that another mediator is involved in the reflex.

It is now clear that the tubulo-glomerular feedback mechanism does play a role in regulating SN GFR. The extent of this role and whether it is the major autoregulatory mechanism have not yet been determined.

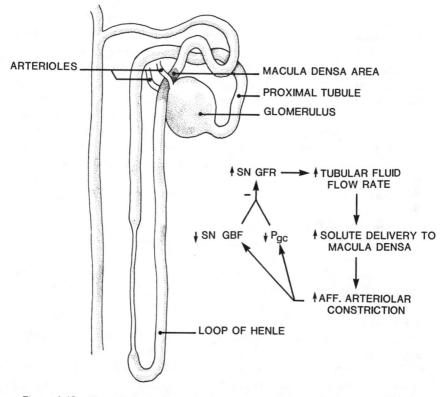

Figure 4-12.   The tubuloglomerular feedback hypothesis. SN GFR = single nephron glomerular filtration rate. P_{gc} = glomerular capillary hydrostatic pressure. SN GBF = single nephron glomerular blood flow rate.

Such a mechanism could play an important role in some pathophysiologic states. For instance, if proximal tubular function is impaired, so that fluid reabsorption occurs at a low rate, the reflex mechanism would reduce GFR and thus limit the loss of fluid from the circulation. This seems to be the case in many of the syndromes of acute renal failure. Injury of tubular cells reduces the rate of reabsorption of filtered salt and water. The resulting rise in the flow rate to the macula densa may signal the glomerulus to reduce GFR. Otherwise, an enormous quantity of salt and water would be lost in the urine.

The ability of the kidney to autoregulate RBF and GFR depends on functioning arterioles. In patients with arteriolar nephrosclerosis, autoregulation is compromised, and relatively minor changes in arterial pressure can lead to large changes in RBF and GFR. This can be of special importance in elderly patients, who usually have some degree of arterial hypertension and arteriosclerosis. Reduction of blood pressure into the normal range in these patients can lead to oliguria or even complete cessation of urine output.

Extrinsic Regulation.

The autoregulatory mechanism or mechanisms control RBF and GFR in the absence of extrinsic neural or humoral influences. However, these extrinsic factors can either override the autoregulatory mechanism or alter its "set point" in many situations. In the recumbent human, renal nerve activity is probably low and there is no extrinsic regulation. A change to the upright position causes a mild vasoconstriction as does exercise in the upright position, but exercise in the recumbent position does not affect RBF or GFR. It has also been observed that changes in the degree of stimulation of arterial baroreceptors cause relatively minor changes in RBF and GFR. These findings suggest that RBF and GFR are altered primarily in response to changes in central blood volume rather than in response to changes in blood pressure. Changes in central blood volume alter the degree of filling of the atria, which is sensed by atrial stretch receptors. It is also known that severe hypoxia reduces RBF and GFR. This results from the stimulation of chemoreceptors in the carotid and aortic bodies.

In sodium depletion, in situations in which cardiac function is compromised, and in hemorrhage, renin release by the kidney and angiotensin formation are stimulated. The increased level of circulating angiotensin reduces RBF to a greater extent than it reduces GFR. In the normal physiologic state, however, there is no strong evidence that angiotensin modulates RBF or GFR. Increased circulating levels of epinephrine also reduce RBF to a greater extent than GFR, and thus, both agents may primarily affect the efferent arteriole.

In situations in which pressor substances, such as epinephrine and angiotensin, are present in greater than normal levels, prostaglandin E_2

production by the kidney is elevated and the vasodilator serves to modulate the effect of the vasoconstrictors.

It should be clear from the foregoing discussion that control of RBF and GFR is a complex and poorly understood subject. A good grasp of the process of autoregulation still eludes us. The roles of angiotensin, dopamine, bradykinin, and prostaglandin are only dimly perceived. Why is it that activation of the sympathetic nervous system by inhibition of atrial stretch receptors has a much greater effect on RBF and GFR than does activation of that system by inhibition of carotid and aortic baroreceptors? What is the role of the parasympathetic, cholinergic nerves? How is it that such diverse substances as acetylcholine, bradykinin, prostaglandin, and angiotensin can reduce the k_f of the glomeruli?

DISTRIBUTION OF RENAL BLOOD FLOW

The highly vascular cortex comprises 75% of the kidney and receives more than 90% of the renal blood flow at a rate of 4 to 5 ml per min per g of tissue. The outer medulla is perfused at a rate of approximately 1.5 ml per min per g. Blood flow through the inner medulla is much less, approximately 0.2 ml per min per g.

Much effort has been expended in attempting to study the distribution of blood flow within the cortex. Initial experimental evidence suggested that a shift in renal blood flow from one section of the cortex to another accompanies alterations in salt and water excretion. For instance, in a dog in which injury of the tricuspid valve reduced cardiac output, measurements indicated that blood flow through the outer cortex decreased and flow through the inner cortex and outer medulla increased. Salt and water retention ensued. When an α-adrenergic blocking agent was administered, the measurements indicated that the distribution of blood flow returned to normal and salt and water excretion was increased. These and other observations led to the suggestion that the shorter nephrons in the outer cortex may have a smaller reabsorptive capacity than do the longer nephrons in the inner cortex, and that changes in the distribution of blood flow and, therefore, the glomerular filtrate between these two populations of nephrons may affect salt excretion and thereby alter body fluid volume. In order to investigate this theory, a variety of techniques were developed to measure changes in the distribution of flow. Among these are measurement of the washout of a bolus injection of an inert, radioactive gas, measurement of local heat clearance, and measurement of the distribution of a bolus injection of glass microspheres labelled with radioisotopes. Unfortunately, these techniques, and even the use of the same technique in different laboratories, have yielded contradictory results. There does not yet seem to be a definitive answer to the question of how and when cortical blood flow may be shifted from one area to another.

BIBLIOGRAPHY

General:

Aukland, K.: Renal Blood Flow. *In* Kidney and Urinary Tract Physiology II. Edited by K. Thurau. International Review of Physiology, Vol. II. Baltimore, University Park Press, 1976.

Navar, L. G.: The Regulation of Glomerular Filtration Rate in Mammalian Kidneys. *In* Physiology of Membrane Disorders. Edited by T. E. Andreoli, J. F. Hoffman, and D. D. Fanestil, New York, Plenum Medical Book Co., 1978.

See also the following chapters from: Brenner, B. M. and Rector, F. C. Jr., (Eds.): The Kidney. Vol. 1. 2nd ed. Philadelphia, W. B. Saunders Co. 1981.

    Chapter 1. Tisher, C. C.: Anatomy of the Kidney.

    Chapter 5. Beeuwkes, R. III, Ichikawa, I., and Brenner, B. M.: The Renal Circulations.

    Chapter 6. Brenner, B. M., Ichikawa, I., and Deen, W. M.: Glomerular Filtration.

Specific:

Aukland, K.: Methods for measuring renal blood flow: total flow and regional distribution. Ann. Rev. Physiol., *42*:543, 1980.

Baer, P. G., and McGiff, John C.: Hormonal systems and renal hemodynamics. Ann. Rev. Physiol., *42*:589, 1980.

Barajas, L.: Anatomy of the juxtaglomerular apparatus. Am. J. Physiol., *237* (Renal Fluid Electrolyte Physiol. 6):F333, 1979.

Beeuwkes, R. III: Vascular organization of the kidney. Ann. Rev. Physiol., *42*:531, 1980.

Blantz, R. C.: Segmental renal vascular resistance: single nephron. Ann. Rev. Physiol., *42*:573, 1980.

Brenner, B. M., Bayliss, C., and Deen, W. M.: Transport of molecules across renal glomerular capillaries. Physiol. Rev., *56*:502, 1976.

Brenner, B. M., Hostetter, T. H., and Humes, H. D.: Glomerular permselectivity: barrier function based on discrimination of molecular size and charge. Am. J. Physiol., *234* (Renal Fluid Electrolyte Physiol. 3):F455, 1978.

Carretero, O. A., and Scicli, A. G.: The renal kallikrein–kinin system. Am. J. Physiol., *238* (Renal Fluid Electrolyte Physiol. 7):F247, 1980.

Navar, L. G.: Renal autoregulation: perspectives from whole kidney and single nephron studies. Am. J. Physiol., *234* (Renal Fluid Electrolyte Physiol. 3):F357, 1978.

Wright, F. S., and Briggs, J. P.: Feedback control of glomerular blood flow, pressure, and filtration rate. Physiol. Rev., *59*:958, 1979.

CHAPTER 5

Tubular Anatomy
and Function

All the remaining chapters of this text deal with various aspects of tubular function and its control. The purpose of this chapter is to describe the microanatomy of the various sections of the nephron, the changes that occur in the composition of the filtrate as it flows through the nephron, and the types of tubular transport mechanisms.

The general anatomic and functional features of epithelial cell layers were described in Chapter 1 (Fig. 1-9). The microanatomy of the renal tubular epithelium varies greatly along the length of the nephron, but each section retains the general features of an epithelial cell system. The cells are arranged in an hexagonal array upon the inner surface of the tubular basement membrane sleeve. They are held together by the zonula occludens, which surrounds each cell near the luminal or apical surface. Except for that junction, the cells are separated from each other by a small distance (~ 300 Å), creating a paracellular space that is essentially the extracellular environment for much of the basolateral membrane. The microanatomy and the transporting properties of the apical and basolateral membranes of each cell differ and it is these differences that permit net transport of various solutes in one direction across the epithelial cell layer to occur.

PROXIMAL TUBULE

Traditionally, the proximal tubule has been considered to be composed of two segments: the convoluted portion, pars convoluta, and the straight portion, pars recta (Fig. 2-2). More recently it has been recognized that the tubule can be divided into at least three segments, S_1, S_2, and S_3, on the basis of subtle anatomic and functional differences that will be described below. S_1 includes the first part of the pars convoluta; S_2, the last part of the pars convoluta and the initial portion of the pars recta; and S_3, the rest of the pars recta. Figure 5-1 is a transmission electron micrograph of the S_1 segment. Note the apical microvilli, the

ZONULA OCCLUDENS ─┐   PARACELLULAR CHANNEL ─┐

BRUSH BORDER ─┐   MITOCHONDRION ─┐

LUMEN

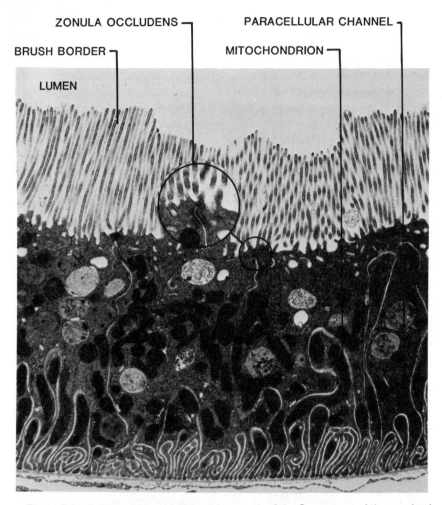

Figure 5-1.   A transmission electron micrograph of the S_1 segment of the proximal tubule of the rabbit. The large circular insert is a higher magnification of the zonula occludens. (Courtesy of Dr. Larry Welling.)

zonula occludens and the evidence of basolateral membrane folding and interdigitation with neighboring cells. Figure 5-2 presents a detailed three-dimensional reconstruction of an average tubular cell from the S_1 segment of the proximal tubule. The surface area of the luminal or apical membrane is extensively multiplied by the presence of the microvilli, which form the brush border of the lumen. Beginning at the zonula occludens (not shown) the basolateral membrane becomes more and more folded as it approaches the basement membrane, and there the individual folds or drapes form fingers that overlie the basement membrane. These folds and fingers greatly multiply the surface area of the

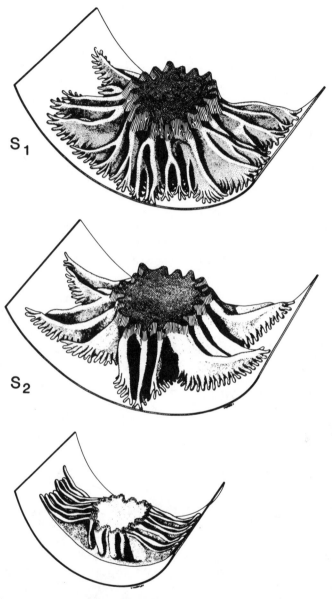

THICK ASCENDING LIMB

Figure 5-2.   Three-dimensional reconstructions of the types of cells found in the S_1 and S_2 segments of the proximal tubule and in the medullary thick ascending limb of the loop of Henle. The relative sizes of the drawings mirror the actual relation of the sizes of these cells in the rabbit nephron. (Courtesy of Drs. Larry and Daniel Welling.)

basolateral membrane. In fact, it has been shown that the surface areas of the luminal and basolateral membranes in this segment are equal.

The folds and fingers of the basolateral membrane of one cell interdigitate with those of neighboring cells so that a constant distance is maintained between the cells. This creates an extensive extracellular or paracellular labyrinth. The small volume of fluid within this labyrinth is in contact with an immensely large surface area of basolateral membrane. It is separated from the luminal fluid by the zonula occludens and from the extracellular fluid surrounding the tubule by the permeable basement membrane sleeve. The exchange of a variety of solutes and water between the cellular and paracellular fluid across the basolateral membrane creates a unique paracellular environment that differs in composition from the luminal and extracellular environments.

Figure 5-3 is a transmission electron micrograph of the S_2 segment. A three-dimensional reconstruction of an average S_2 cell is shown in Figure 5-2. The height of the brush border is less than in an S_1 cell and the basolateral membrane is not as extensively folded. Still, the areas of the apical membrane and the basolateral membrane are equal in this

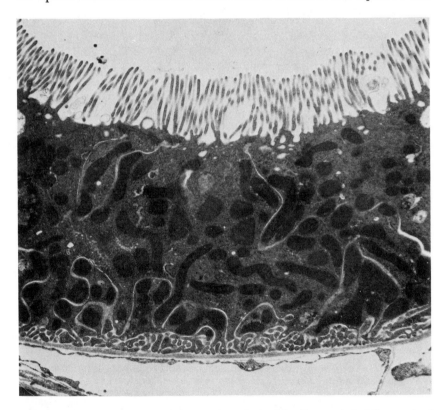

Figure 5-3.   A transmission electron micrograph of the S_2 segment of the proximal tubule of the rabbit. (Courtesy of Dr. Larry Welling.)

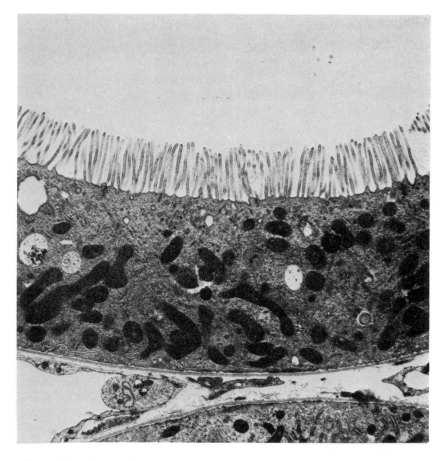

Figure 5-4. A transmission electron micrograph of the S_3 segment of the proximal tubule of the rabbit. (Courtesy of Dr. Larry Welling.)

segment. In the S_3 segment (Fig. 5-4), the brush border is also extensive, but the basolateral folds are poorly developed. Thus, the apical surface area exceeds the basolateral area.

Much of our information regarding proximal tubular function comes from in vivo micropuncture experiments performed mainly on amphibia and rats and from in vitro studies of isolated segments of rabbit tubules. The rat micropuncture experiments have been limited to the pars convoluta and most of the studies of the isolated segments have concentrated on S_1 and S_2. Investigation of the function of the S_3 segment has been limited.

The complexity of the structure of the proximal tubular cells is mirrored by the variety of physiologic tasks they perform. The proximal tubule reabsorbs 60 to 70% of the salt and water in the glomerular filtrate. All the filtered glucose is normally reabsorbed here. Amino

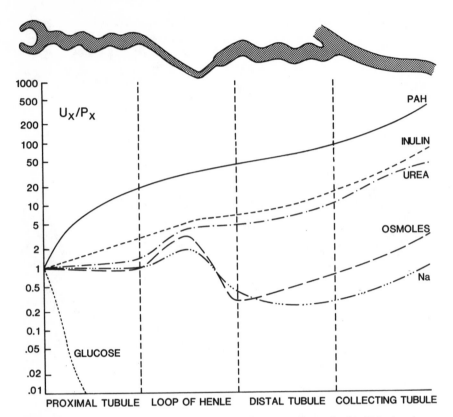

Figure 5-5. Changes in the urine to plasma concentration ratio (U_x/P_x) of various substances along the length of the nephron. Note that the ordinate is a log scale.

acids, urea, bicarbonate, phosphate, potassium, and calcium are reabsorbed to varying extents. A variety of organic acids and bases, including many substances foreign to the body, are secreted into the tubular fluid by these cells, as are hydrogen ions and ammonia. To a large degree, the three different segments of the proximal tubule possess similar transport mechanisms. The major functional differences that have been discovered so far are in rates of transport rather than in types.

The proximal tubule is highly permeable to water. This is at least partially a reflection of the tremendous membrane surface area. Because of this high hydraulic permeability or conductance, a large volume of the filtered water can be reabsorbed by the generation of small osmotic pressure gradients. The tubular epithelium is also permeable to small electrolytes, resulting in a high electrical conductance. The high conductance pathway is between cells, through the zonula occludens and the paracellular space. The individual cell membranes are much less conductive. The high conductance of the paracellular path prevents the establishment of large differences in the concentration of small ions across the tubular wall by active transport of the ions or by water reabsorption. The low conductance of the cell membrane, however, does permit large differences in electrical potential and in ion concentrations to be established between the cellular and tubular or extracellular fluid.

The reabsorption of a major part of the filtrate is accomplished primarily by two forces: the Na-K-ATPase system, which transports Na from the cell to the paracellular space, and the colloid osmotic pressure of the blood in the peritubular capillaries. Together, these forces, in concert with the physical properties of the tubule and other ancillary transport systems, reabsorb 60 to 70% of the filtrate without detectably altering the osmotic concentration of the tubular fluid. Only minor changes in the concentration of most of the inorganic ions occur.

Figure 5-5 illustrates the changes that occur in the composition of the tubular fluid as it flows through the proximal tubule. Figure 5-6 illustrates the fraction of the filtered *amount* remaining in the tubular fluid. Since inulin is filtered but neither reabsorbed nor secreted, its concentration changes only as water is reabsorbed, and it increases by a factor

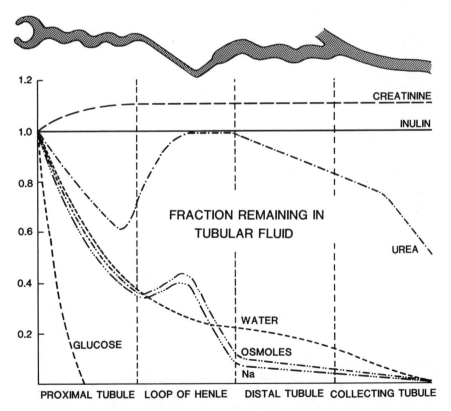

Figure 5-6. Changes in the fraction of the filtered amount of substances remaining in the tubular fluid along the length of the nephron $((U_x/P_x)/(U_{in}/P_{in}))$.

of 2.5 to 3.3 as 60 to 70% of the water is reabsorbed. The total solute or osmotic concentration does not change, indicating that 60 to 70% of the filtered solute is also reabsorbed. The Na concentration does not change and only minor changes occur in the concentration of the principal inorganic anions; the Cl concentration rises slightly and the HCO_3 concentration falls to some extent. All the filtered glucose and amino acids are usually reabsorbed within the first third of the proximal tubule. Urea also is reabsorbed in the proximal tubule. Since its rate of reabsorption is less than the rate for water, its concentration rises somewhat. The changes in para-aminohippurate (PAH) concentration are illustrated in Figure 5-5 as an example of substances that are filtered and secreted. The rise in concentration in the tubular fluid is the sum of two processes: reabsorption of water and the active addition of the solute to the tubular fluid by the tubular cells.

LOOP OF HENLE

At the end of the S_3 segment of the proximal tubule, a sudden transition in cell type occurs as the proximal tubule ends and the thin segment of the loop of Henle begins. In the long juxtamedullary nephrons, the transition occurs in the outer medulla and marks the boundary between the inner and outer stripes of the outer medulla. The cells of the thin limb are relatively flat except where the nucleus causes the cell to bulge into the lumen (Fig. 5-7). There are few microvilli on the apical surface, but the basolateral membrane does interdigitate with neighboring cells to some extent. The mitochondria are small and few in number.

The function of the thin limb of the loop of Henle has been studied by in vivo micropuncture experiments on animals, such as the hamster, which have papilla that extend into the ureter and by in vitro perfusion of isolated segments taken from the rabbit kidney. The descending limb is highly permeable to water, which moves passively across the tubular wall when an osmotic gradient exists between the tubular fluid and the interstitial fluid. In the medullary region, the loop of Henle descends into an interstitial environment that is increasingly hypertonic as the papilla is approached. The reabsorption of water in response to this gradient raises the osmotic concentration of the tubular fluid as it flows deeper into the medulla. This is reflected by a rise in total solute and inulin concentrations (Fig. 5-5). No known active transport processes exist in the thin descending limb. The degree of permeability of the tubular epithelium to salt and urea, two major constituents of the medullary interstitial fluid, is a controversial issue. Net addition of salt and urea to the tubular contents may occur.

In those nephrons that have a thin ascending limb, some minor anatomic differences exist between the descending and ascending segments. In some species at least, the cells in the ascending limb have no microvilli and the basolateral interdigitations are greatly reduced. There are also functional differences. The ascending limb has a much lower permeability to water and loses solute by a poorly understood mechanism, so that the osmotic concentration of the tubular fluid is reduced below that of the surrounding interstitium.

At the juncture of the thin and thick segments of the ascending limb of the loop of Henle, the tubular cells become cuboidal and more complex in shape (Fig. 5-7). The basolateral membrane is deeply enfolded, and projections of the cell extend some distance circumferentially to interdigitate with neighboring cells and form complex paracellular channels that open onto the basement membrane (Fig. 5-2). The cytoplasm within these folds contains many large, elongated mitochondria.

The function of the thick segment of the loop of Henle has been directly studied only by in vitro perfusion of isolated segments. The thick segment of the loop, like the thin ascending limb, has a low permeability to water; its conductance or permeability to small ions is also relatively small. However, the thick segment actively reabsorbs Na

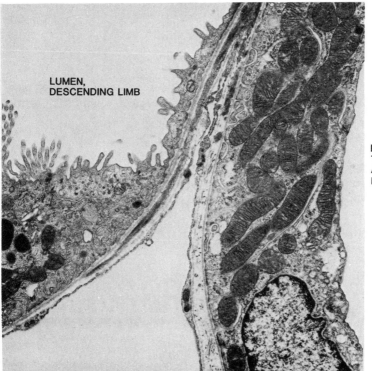

Figure 5-7. An electron micrograph of two structures found in the medulla of the rabbit. On the left is a segment of a cell from the thin descending limb of Henle's loop. The epithelium is thin except in the region where the nucleus (not shown) is found. On the right is a segment of the thick ascending limb. Note the large elongated mitochondria. (Courtesy of Dr. Larry Welling.)

and Cl. This segment of the nephron is often called the diluting segment, because the removal of salt with little water from the tubular contents dilutes the salt and the osmotic concentration of the tubular fluid (Fig. 5-5). The addition of the reabsorbed Na and Cl with little water to the medullary interstitial fluid compartment raises the osmotic and salt concentration of that compartment. Potassium is also reabsorbed by the thick ascending limb.

DISTAL TUBULE

The distal convoluted tubule is usually considered to begin at the point of contact of the nephron with the juxtaglomerular apparatus and to end at the point where it joins with another distal tubule or a collecting tubule. Traditionally, the distal tubule has also been considered to be a distinct functional unit of the nephron. Recent research, however, has blurred that distinction. Both anatomically and functionally, the distal tubule seems to be a zone of transition between the diluting segment and the cortical collecting tubule.

Cells in the early part of the distal tubule closely resemble those in the ascending limb (Fig. 5-8). The peritubular surfaces are deeply enfolded and the cytoplasm contains many large mitochondria. In the late segments of the distal tubule, the cells resemble those in the cortical sections of the collecting tubule (Fig. 5-9). This segment has recently been designated the initial collecting tubule. The deep basolateral folds and interdigitations with neighboring cells are not present and the number and size of the mitochondria are decreased. A "mid-segment," now called the connecting tubule, can be distinguished from both the early and late segments.

Our knowledge of the function of the distal tubule has come almost entirely from micropuncture studies performed on the rat. The initial segments of the distal tubule are relatively impermeable to water. The late segment, at least in some species, responds to antidiuretic hormone, so that its water permeability is high in the presence of the hormone and low in its absence. The conductance of the distal tubular epithelium to small ions is much less than that of the proximal tubule, so the reabsorptive mechanisms for Na and Cl are opposed by only small back-fluxes. This, in combination with a low rate of water reabsorption, enables the transport mechanisms to establish large concentration gradients between the tubular lumen and the interstitial fluid (low U/P ratios, Fig. 5-5). Despite this, only a small fraction of the filtered amount of solute and water is reabsorbed in the distal tubule (Fig. 5-6).

Potassium can be reabsorbed and secreted here. Hydrogen and ammonia secretion and bicarbonate reabsorption continue, but there is little transport of organic substances. This segment of the nephron also has a low permeability to urea, so any water reabsorption that occurs increases the tubular fluid concentration of that substance (Fig. 5-5) and

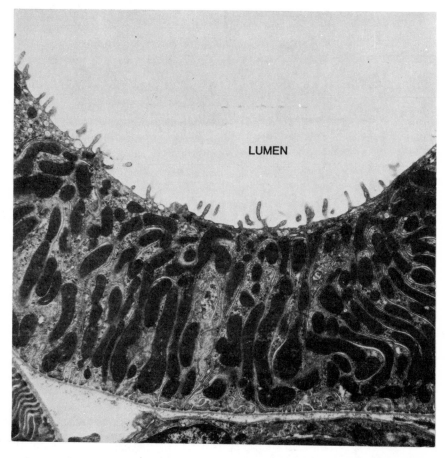

LUMEN

Figure 5-8. A transmission electron micrograph of the initial segment of the distal tubule of the rabbit. Note the extensive interdigitation of neighboring cells and the large number of mitochondria. (Courtesy of Dr. Larry Welling.)

any other to which the tubule is impermeable (such as PAH). The adrenocortical hormone, aldosterone, stimulates both sodium reabsorption and potassium secretion in the distal tubule.

COLLECTING TUBULE

Two cell types are found in the walls of the collecting tubule (Fig. 5-9). The principal cell, often called the "light cell" occurs in greater numbers than the intercalated or "dark" cell. The major features that distinguish the two in the transmission electron micrograph are the densely stained cytoplasm and the large number of mitochondria and other cellular organelles found in the intercalated cells. Closer examination reveals other differences. A single long cilium projects into the lumen from the apical membrane of the principal cell (Fig. 5-10). This cell also has short,

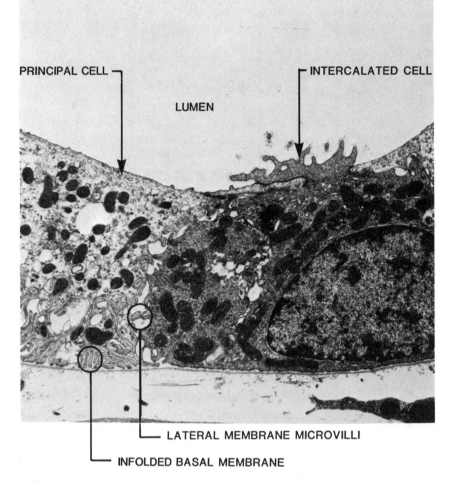

Figure 5-9.   A transmission electron micrograph of a segment of the cortical collecting tubule of the rabbit. A principal or "light" cell appears on the right and an intercalated or "dark" cell on the left. (Courtesy of Dr. Larry Welling.)

blunt microvilli protruding into the lumen, whereas the intercalated cells have more prominent ridges on the apical surface which, in cross section in a transmission electron micrograph, appear as microvilli that are longer than those on the light cells (Fig. 5-9). Small microvillous projections appear on the lateral surfaces of both of these cuboidal cells, which seem to interlock with projections from neighboring cells. Unlike the cells in other sections of the nephron, the basal membranes of these cells are distinct from the lateral membranes. The basal membrane has the appearance of a mesa with tortuous "canyons" that penetrate deeply into the body of the cell. These are much more extensive in the principal cells than in the dark cells. The functional significance of architectural

PRINCIPAL CELL ⌐   ⌐ INTERCALATED CELL

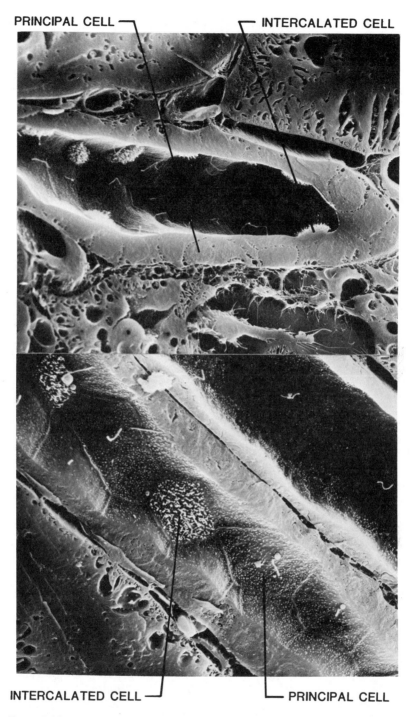

INTERCALATED CELL ⌐   ⌐ PRINCIPAL CELL

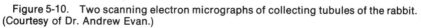

Figure 5-10.   Two scanning electron micrographs of collecting tubules of the rabbit.
(Courtesy of Dr. Andrew Evan.)

features of the apical, lateral, and basal membranes of these cells is unknown. Neither do we know precisely what differences in function may exist between the two cell types. As the collecting tubule descends into the medulla toward the papilla, the cells become more columnar and the number of intercalated cells decreases.

Studies of the function of the collecting tubule, particularly the cortical sections, have been performed almost entirely by in vitro perfusion of isolated segments. Some information on the function of the papillary segments has been derived from micropuncture experiments and from experiments in which small catheters have been threaded into individual ducts.

ADH controls the water permeability of the collecting tubule throughout its length. In the presence of the hormone, the hypotonic tubular fluid entering the cortical sections of the collecting tubule loses water and its osmotic concentration rises to equal that of the filtrate. In the medulla, the high osmotic concentration of the interstitium provides a force for continued water reabsorption, and the osmotic concentration of the tubular fluid continues to increase along the length of the tubule.

Sodium and chloride are reabsorbed by the collecting tubule, and the transport of sodium is stimulated by aldosterone. Potassium, hydrogen, and ammonium are also transported by the collecting tubules. The conductance of the epithelium to small ions is low. Thus, in the cortical sections of the collecting tubule, the concentration of Na and Cl may continue to drop if ADH is absent and little water is reabsorbed. When ADH is present, the rate of water reabsorption exceeds the rate of solute reabsorption and the concentration of Na and Cl rises.

In the medullary sections of the collecting tubule, the rate of solute transport is low, but the resulting changes in urine concentration are great because only a small fraction of the filtered solute reaches the collecting tubule and because water reabsorption can vary so greatly.

The cortical and outer medullary sections of the collecting tubule are relatively impermeable to urea so the concentration increases as water is reabsorbed. However, urea is reabsorbed by the inner medullary section of the tubule and enters the medullary interstitium, where it participates in establishing a high osmotic concentration.

SUMMARY

The anatomically complex cells of the permeable proximal tubule reabsorb the greater mass of the filtrate and transport a large variety of organic and inorganic substances, without causing any changes in the osmotic concentration of the tubular fluid. Only minor changes in the concentrations of the major ions occur. The electrolyte and water reabsorptive systems in the proximal tubule can be classified as high capacity, low gradient systems. The anatomy of the medulla and the transport characteristics of the loop of Henle permit the establishment of a hypertonic environment in the medulla, which in turn, osmotically concentrates the urine in the collecting ducts. The more impermeable distal tubule and collecting duct reabsorb smaller fractions of the filtered water and solute than does the proximal tubule, but under the influence of hormones and other factors, they can vary the ratio of salt to water in the reabsorbed fluid. Thus, the osmotic concentration and the concentration of individual solutes in the final urine can vary over a wide range. The electrolyte and water transport systems in the distal tubule and collecting tubule, in contrast to the proximal tubule, are low capacity, high gradient systems. Almost all the tubular transport mechanisms are regulated in such a way as to minimize any changes that may occur in the volume of the organism's extracellular fluid, its osmotic concentration, the concentration of its major solutes, and its acid-base status.

ELECTRICAL PROPERTIES OF THE NEPHRON

The movement of ions across membranes can be strongly influenced by gradients of electrical potential. In the nephron, the reabsorption and secretion of a variety of ions are affected by electrical gradients across the individual cell membranes and also across the entire tubular wall. A knowledge of these electrical properties is essential to a full understanding of the transport mechanisms.

The interior of most tubular cells is negative with respect to both the interstitial fluid surrounding the tubule and the tubular fluid. This electrical gradient across the apical and basolateral membranes favors the movement of cations into the cell and the movement of anions out. Since the molecular composition and transport properties of the two membranes differ, the electrical potential difference (V) across each membrane could be different if the ISF and the tubular fluid were electrically insulated from each other. In that situation, an electrical potential difference of some magnitude could exist across the cell layer between the lumen and ISF (a transepithelial potential difference, V_t). However, if there is a low resistance (high conductance) connection between the tubular fluid and the interstitial fluid, such as the paracellular pathway, it could serve as an electrical shunt between the two fluids and maintain V_t at a low level.

A diagram of the two situations is presented in Figure 5-11. An electrical circuit diagram is superimposed on the drawing of a tubular cell. The transport properties of each cell membrane are represented in the expanded boxes by a battery and a resistor in series. The two membranes are connected to each other through the cell by a very low resistance path, the intracellular fluid, and by a parallel circuit through the paracellular shunt path that includes a resistance element, the zonula occludens. The three microelectrodes illustrated are used to measure the electrical potential difference between the interior of the cell and the

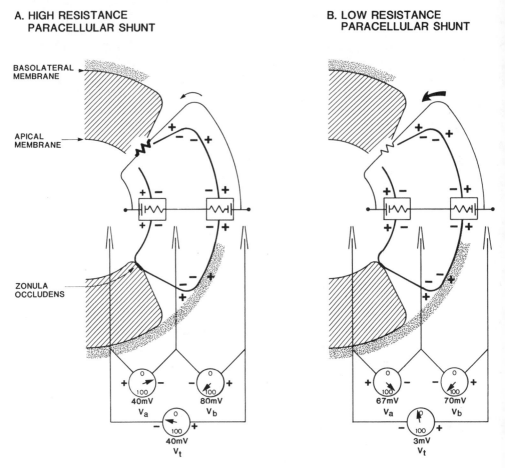

A. HIGH RESISTANCE PARACELLULAR SHUNT

B. LOW RESISTANCE PARACELLULAR SHUNT

Figure 5-11. A diagram of hypothetical tubular segments showing how high and low paracellular shunt resistances may affect the measured transmembrane and trans-epithelial voltage.

interstitial fluid (V_b), between the cell and the tubular fluid (V_a), and between the tubular fluid and interstitial fluid (V_t).

In the hypothetical situation depicted in A, the basolateral membrane establishes a potential difference (V_b) between the cellular fluid and the interstitial fluid of 80 mV, the interior of the cell negative with respect to the interstitial fluid. The differing properties of the apical membrane permit it to establish a potential difference (V_a) between the cell interior and the tubular fluid of 40 mV, cell negative. If the shunt resistance is large, as in A, then a large voltage drop could occur between the interstitial fluid and the tubular fluid, even though the actual current flow might be small. In A, that voltage (V_t) is 40 mV, tubular fluid negative with respect to the interstitial fluid. A small current flow through the large shunt resistance in A would have only a small effect on the voltages generated across the two cell membranes (V_a and V_b).

If the shunt resistance were low, as in B, even a very large current flow would produce only a small voltage difference between tubular fluid and the interstitial fluid. In the example shown in B, V_t equals 3 mV, tubular fluid negative. Although a large current flow through the paracellular shunt in B would produce only a small V_t, it has other significant effects. Current flow from the ISF to the tubular fluid tends to depolarize the basolateral membrane and polarize the apical membrane. In this hypothetical example, V_b has fallen to 70 mV and V_a has risen to 67 mV. The actual degree of the influence of the shunt current on these voltages depends on the properties of the individual membranes.

Some additional comments can be made in regard to the hypothetical situations portrayed in Figure 5-11. The current flow through the paracellular shunt could be carried by cations moving into the tubular fluid or anions moving out of the tubular fluid. It is important to realize that the simple batteries and resistors used to illustrate membrane properties represent the sum of the products of chemical gradients and fractional conductances for several ions (see Equation 1-9), plus the possible contribution of electrogenic transport mechanisms. The tubular fluid is indicated to be negative with respect to the interstitial fluid. However, in some areas of the nephron, that electrical potential gradient can be reversed, evidently as a result of changes in the properties of either cell membrane or both. Since V_a, V_b, and V_t at any point along the tubule are largely the result of ionic concentration gradients, alterations in the composition of tubular fluid and in the rates of membrane transport can result in changes in the magnitude of these voltages.

In the proximal tubule, the paracellular shunt resistance is small and, even though large fluxes of ions can occur through that path, V_t is small. In the earliest segments of the proximal tubule, V_t is on the order of 2 to 4 mV, lumen negative. In later segments, V_t is oriented in the opposite direction but the magnitude is about the same. In the thick ascending limb, the paracellular shunt resistance is somewhat greater than in the proximal tubule and V_t equals 4 to 10 mV, tubular fluid positive. At a point midway along the length of the distal tubule of some species, V_t abruptly changes to about 30 to 50 mV, tubular fluid negative. The mechanisms responsible for this change are not known. The paracellular shunt resistance is much greater, however, than in the proximal tubule. The electrical properties of the collecting tubule are even more bewildering. The paracellular shunt resistance is large, but V_t evidently can vary over a wide range in both directions from zero. This may occur as a result of changes in tubular fluid composition or in the plasma levels of aldosterone.

TYPES OF TUBULAR TRANSPORT MECHANISMS

Solutes cross the tubular epithelium by a large variety of transport mechanisms. We shall attempt to describe here the general types of transport processes that occur in the tubule (See Chapter 1).

Passive Diffusion

The most simple type of transport that can occur is passive diffusion; that is, random movement of an ion or molecule driven by the thermal energy it possesses.There is no direct interaction with other solutes or with components of the cell membranes. Net movement across the tubular epithelium by diffusion occurs if a concentration gradient for an uncharged solute exists. The net rate of movement is determined by the magnitude of the gradient and the permeability of the epithelium to that solute (Equation 1-1). Initially, no gradients exist between the glomerular filtrate entering the tubule and the interstitial fluid surrounding the nephron, except protein, to which the tubular epithelium is impermeable. As the filtrate flows along the tubule, active transport mechanisms begin to establish osmotic and chemical gradients and the reabsorption of water contributes to the formation of chemical gradients. The reabsorption of urea in the proximal tubule is an example of transport by passive diffusion. As water is reabsorbed from the filtrate, the urea concentration rises, creating a chemical gradient that drives net diffusion in the reabsorptive direction.

If a solute is charged, net movement across the membranes will result if either an electrical or concentration gradient or both exist. Again, the rate and direction of transport are determined by the magnitude of the combined electrochemical gradient and the conductance of the epithelium to that solute (Equation 1-8). For ions, the route of least resistance or greatest conductance for passive diffusion in response to these gradients is across the zonula occludens and through the paracellular pathway. A smaller amount may diffuse through the cell membranes.

Passive Transport of Weak Electrolytes

Chemical gradients for passive diffusion of certain substances can be established by alterations in the pH of tubular fluid. Weak organic acids and bases with pK values in the range 3.5 to 9.5 may have two forms in tubular fluid. The nonionized forms of these substances are much more lipid-soluble than the ionized forms and can more easily diffuse through the tubular wall. The direction and magnitude of the diffusion gradient of the nonionized form across the tubular wall depends on the direction and magnitude of the hydrogen ion concentration gradient and the pK of the substance.

Let us first consider how this applies to weak bases (Fig. 5-12). In acidic tubular fluid, their reaction with hydrogen ions ($B + H^+ \rightleftarrows BH^+$) is shifted towards formation of the charged, lipid-insoluble form. Passive reabsorption of the substance is suppressed because this poorly permeant form cannot readily diffuse out across the tubular epithelium and thus is trapped in the urine. Passive secretion from the blood to tubular fluid is favored because the nonionized, lipid-soluble form exists in higher concentration in the relatively alkaline blood than it

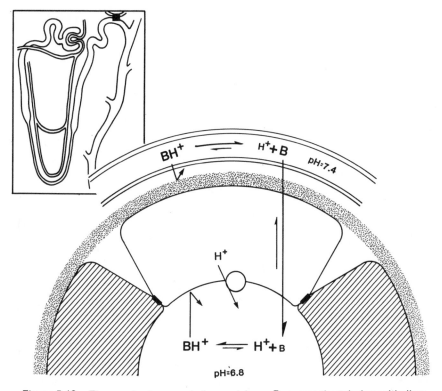

Figure 5-12.   The passive transport of a weak base, B, across the tubular epithelium as a result of a difference in pH between peritubular blood and tubular fluid.

does in acidic tubular fluid. When this form diffuses into the tubular fluid, it is titrated to BH^+ and the low concentration of the diffusible form in tubular fluid is maintained. In this manner, the excretion of weak bases is increased when the urine is made acid. Conversely, if the tubular fluid is alkaline, reabsorption is enhanced, secretion is slowed, and the rate of excretion falls. Ammonium is a prime example of a weak base that is passively transported (see Chapter 10). Other examples are quinine, quinicrine, chloroquine, neutral red, and procaine.

The reaction of weak acids with hydrogen ($A^- + H^+ \rightleftarrows HA$) is shifted towards formation of the nonionized, lipid-soluble form in acidic tubular fluid, so reabsorption is favored and secretion is suppressed. The excretion of salicylic acid, phenobarbitol, and nitrofurantoin are affected in this manner.

Carrier-Mediated Transport

Carrier-mediated transport has been described in detail in Chapter 1. One example of a carrier-mediated transport system in the nephron is the mechanism that reabsorbs glucose from the glomerular filtrate. This mechanism exhibits the three distinguishing characteristics of carrier-mediated transport: specificity, competition, and saturation. It will transport only a small number of carbohydrates with similar structures: xylose, fructose, and galactose, as well as glucose. All four of these substances compete with each other for attachment to the carrier molecule. However, the transport system has a higher affinity for glucose than for the other three. The rate of glucose reabsorption increases as the concentration in the glomerular filtrate rises up to about 3.75 mg/ml. Any increment in concentration above that level results only in excretion of glucose; reabsorption increases no further (see Fig. 3-5).

If the tubular wall is permeable to some degree to the transported substance, an additional limitation is placed on the rate of transport, since the substance can diffuse back in the opposite direction down the concentration gradient established by the pump. This is not important in the case of glucose because the tubular wall is only slightly permeable to it. It diffuses down its concentration gradient from the blood back into the tubular lumen at only a very slow rate. An example of a "pump-leak" or gradient-limited system in which the concentration gradient does play an important role in limiting the net rate of transport is the active reabsorption of Na by the nephron. As the active transport system removes Na from the tubular fluid, the concentration falls and a chemical gradient for passive diffusion back into the tubular lumen is established. The larger the gradient, the greater the rate of "leakage" of Na back into the tubule. There is a limiting maximum gradient at which the passive back flux into the lumen equals the active flux out and no further net transport can take place. Active transport mechanisms in the nephron fall into one of these two types: those shown to have a relatively fixed maximum rate of transport, that is, capacity-limited systems such as that for glucose; and those limited more by the concentration gradient they can establish than by the maximum rate of the pump, that is, gradient-limited systems.

Let us consider in more detail some of the factors affecting the passive back-flux in a gradient-limited transport system. The magnitude of the chemical gradient driving the passive back-flux is affected not only by the rate of the active forward flux but also by reabsorption of water. If the rate of water reabsorption is high, then the active reabsorption of an ion such as Na produces little change in the tubular fluid Na concentration. The gradient for passive back-flux is low and the net rate of Na reabsorption is relatively high.

Such is the case in the proximal tubule. The rate of reabsorption of water is usually as fast as the rate of Na transport, little or no gradient for passive back-flux exists, and despite the high conductance of the epithelium to Na, the net rate of Na reabsorption is high. If the rate of water reabsorption is slowed, active Na reabsorption begins to reduce the tubular fluid concentration. The passive back-flux of Na then rises to approach the rate of the active flux. Thus the rate of *net* reabsorption is reduced.

The tubular fluid flow rate also affects the net transport of an ion by a gradient-limited mechanism. If, for instance, the flow rate is low in the distal tubule, the supply of Na to the pump is low and it quickly lowers the concentration to a point where the passive back-flux rate severely limits further net transport. If the flow rate is high, the supply of Na to the pump is constantly replenished and the concentration in the tubular fluid is maintained at a higher level. This limits the rate of the back-flux and consequently the *net* rate of reabsorption is higher. To summarize, a high rate of water reabsorption and a high tubular fluid flow rate limit the establishment of chemical gradients, and thereby, can potentially increase the rate of reabsorption by gradient-limited active transport mechanisms. A profitable exercise for the student would be to consider the effect of varying rates of water reabsorption and tubular fluid flow on the net rate of secretion of solutes such as K and H by gradient-limited mechanisms.

Cotransport Systems

In the nephron as well as in other epithelia, there are several membrane "cotransport" systems, in which the transport of one substance is coupled to another. In some cases the movement of one substance down its electrochemical gradient is used to drive the movement of another substance. For instance, in the luminal membrane of the proximal tubule, a carrier molecule facilitates the movement of Na and glucose from the lumen into the cell. Both substances are required in the tubular fluid to activate the carrier. The electrochemical gradient for Na between the tubular fluid and the cytoplasm actually causes the inward movement of both glucose and Na. The Na gradient is maintained by the Na pump (Na-K-ATPase) in the basolateral membrane. Thus, the Na-glucose transport is a "secondary" active transport system. This cotransport system is called a "symport." Another symport system is a coupled NaCl transport mechanism, which moves Na and Cl from the lumen into the cell in some sections of the nephron. There may also be "antiport" systems, in which two ions of the same charge are exchanged across a membrane. The Na-K-ATPase system is one example of an antiport mechanism.

BIBLIOGRAPHY

General:

Burg, M. B.: Renal Handling of Sodium, Chloride, Water, Amino Acids, and Glucose. *In* The Kidney. 2nd ed. Edited by B. M. Brenner, and F. C. Rector, Jr. Philadelphia, W. B. Saunders Co., 1981.

Tisher, C. C.: Anatomy of the Kidney. *In* The Kidney. 2nd ed. Edited by B. M. Brenner, and F. C. Rector, Jr. Philadelphia, W. B. Saunders Co., 1981.

Specific:

Boulpaep, E. L.: Electrical phenomena in the nephron. Kidney Internat. 9:88, 1976.

Fromter, E.: Electrophysiology and Isotonic Fluid Reabsorption of Proximal Tubules of Mammalian Nephrons. *In* Kidney and Urinary Tract Physiology. Edited by K. Thurau. Physiology, Series 1. Vol. 6. MTP International Review of Science. Baltimore, University Park Press, 1974.

Milne, M. D., Scribner, B. H., and Crawford, M.A.: Non-Ionic diffusion and the excretion of weak acids and bases. Am. J. Med., 24:709, 1958.

Sachs, G.: Ion pumps in the renal tubule. Am. J. Physiol., 233 (Renal Fluid Electrolyte Physiol. 2): F359, 1977.

Valtin, H.: Structural and functional heterogeneity of mammalian nephrons. Am. J. Physiol., 233 (Renal Fluid Electrolyte Physiol. 2): F491, 1977.

Welling, D. J., and Welling, L. W.: Cell shape as an indicator of volume reabsorption in proximal nephron. Fed. Proc. 38:121, 1979.

CHAPTER *6*

Excretion of
Organic Molecules

The kidneys efficiently retain filtered glucose and amino acids but eliminate a variety of other organic substances from the body, most of which are metabolites derived from endogenous or exogenous sources. Urea, a nonpolar by-product of protein catabolism, is the most abundant organic constituent in the urine. Most other organic substances exist principally as anions or cations in plasma and urine. The renal tubules have evolved rather specialized mechanisms for excreting these substances.

UREA

Urea is eliminated from the body principally by the kidneys. The amount of urea excreted in the urine is primarily dependent on the amount of nitrogen ingested in the diet. Urea is present in the plasma at a concentration of 18 to 36 mg/dl, averaging about 27 mg/dl, or 4.5 mM. Clinically, however, its concentration is usually expressed as the concentration of "urea nitrogen," the normal range being 9 to 18 mg/dl (blood urea nitrogen, BUN). Urea diffuses into all body water compartments, but the rate of diffusion across capillary and cell membranes differs from organ to organ.

Urea is freely filtered by the glomerulus, but its rate of clearance from plasma is less than that of inulin since it is reabsorbed at various sites along the renal tubule (Chapters 5 and 7). The rate of reabsorption and thus the clearance from plasma is highly dependent on the rate of urine flow. With extreme dehydration and oliguria (urine flow less than 400 ml/24 hours), the urea clearance falls precipitously and the plasma level rises. By contrast, in polyuric states the urea clearance increases, causing the plasma urea level to decrease. The dependence of urea clearance on urine flow rate is explained by the fact that the reabsorption of urea by passive diffusion from urine to blood is dependent on the concentration of the solute in the tubular fluid. Water reabsorption exceeds the rate of urea diffusion. This increases the tubular fluid urea concentration, which then raises the rate of urea diffusion into the interstitium. Consequently, the rate of reabsorption depends on two important factors: (1) the absolute rate of water absorption and (2) the tubule fluid flow rate. For instance, high rates of water reabsorption in the proximal tubule increase the tubule fluid urea level and the rate of urea reabsorption. Conversely, if proximal tubular water reabsorption is reduced, the urea concentration and the rate of urea reabsorption remains low. The high flow rate of fluid with a low concentration of urea into the rest of the nephron also depresses urea reabsorption distally. In general, factors that depress water reabsorption and increase the tubular fluid flow rate reduce urea reabsorption and increase excretion, thereby enhancing the clearance of urea from the plasma (Fig. 6-1). Factors that increase water reabsorption or reduce tubular fluid flow increase urea reabsorption and tend to promote urea retention.

Recent studies indicate that urea may be actively secreted into the urine by the pars recta of the proximal tubule. The quantitative significance of urea secretion is not firmly established, although it appears that some humans may lack this secretory component and have plasma urea levels higher than normal despite a normal glomerular filtration rate.

The renal tubules have segments that are either highly permeable or relatively impermeable to urea. Because of this fact, urea can freely diffuse out of the urine in some tubule segments but not in others. The proximal tubules and the medullary collecting tubules are relatively permeable to urea, those segments in between being less permeable. Urea that is passively absorbed by the medullary collecting system enters the interstitium and the vasa recta, which in turn, promotes its accumulation to high levels in the medullary interstitium through the countercurrent process (see Chapter 7 and Fig. 7-10). The high concentration of urea in the medullary interstitial fluid is thought to promote water loss from the descending limb of the loop of Henle. According to one current theory, the descending limb may be relatively impermeable to NaCl. Thus, the loss of water would increase the NaCl concentration of tubular fluid above that in the interstitium. The theory then predicts that the thin ascending limb of Henle's loop, which is impermeable to water, is also slightly permeable to urea and highly permeable to NaCl. This would permit NaCl to diffuse out at a faster rate than urea enters. Thus, the higher concentration of urea in the interstitium than in the tubule fluid may indirectly cause the reabsorption of NaCl without water, thereby diluting the ascending limb tubule fluid in relation to the interstitium (see Chapter 7). Whether this theory is correct or not, it is clear that urea plays an important role in the generation of a dilute urine in the ascending limb and a concentrated urine in the collecting system.

In patients with renal failure, glomerular filtration is greatly reduced and urea accumulates in the plasma to high levels (100 to 200 mg/dl).

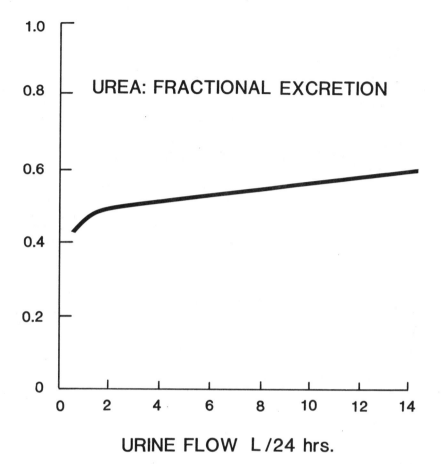

Figure 6-1. The effect of changes in urine flow rate on the fractional excretion of urea.

It was one of the first chemicals identified in the plasma of patients who were desperately ill due to renal failure, and clinicians still refer to this condition as "uremia." Recent evidence indicates that urea is not especially toxic and that the clinical syndrome of uremia is due to other substances inadequately excreted by patients with renal failure.

ORGANIC ANIONS

PAH

The organic anion secretory mechanism has been studied extensively. Hippurate, a natural organic anion, and the first peptide to be synthesized by chemists, and its para-amino derivative (PAH) are eliminated from the body by this means. (Fig. 6-2). Some organic anions are extensively but reversibly bound to plasma proteins, especially at low en-

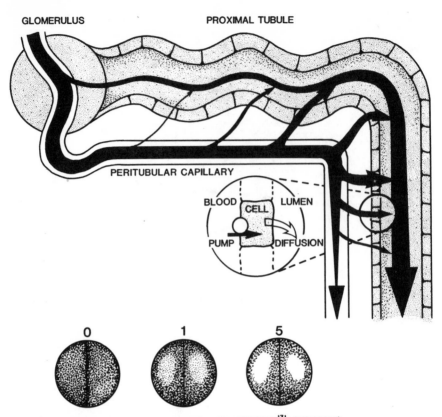

GLOMERULUS   PROXIMAL TUBULE

PERITUBULAR CAPILLARY

BLOOD   LUMEN
CELL

PUMP   DIFFUSION

0   1   5

TIME AFTER INTRAVENOUS INJECTION OF HIPPURAN[131]I (MINUTES)

Figure 6-2. The proximal tubular secretion of hippurate (Hippuran-^{131}I). The three circles represent oscilloscope images of radioactive emissions from the kidneys.

dogenous levels. Consequently, they are not filtered to a great extent by the glomerulus. As the blood flows out of the glomerulus past the proximal tubules, the free organic anions in peritubular plasma are secreted into the urine. The secretory process lowers the concentration of free organic anion in the plasma, thereby causing most of the anion bound to plasma proteins to be "unloaded." In this way, substances that cannot be filtered because they are bound to plasma proteins may be virtually eliminated from the blood in one passage through the renal cortex.

The efficient extraction of many organic anions from the blood is due to an interesting arrangement of cellular transport units in the proximal tubule. The free anion diffusing out of the capillary binds to a transporter located within the basolateral plasma membrane (see inset in Fig. 6-2). This transporter shifts the anion into the cytoplasm and elevates the cytoplasmic concentration to a level many times greater than that in the plasma. Since the luminal membrane of the cell is much more permeable to the organic anion than the peritubular membrane, the anion diffuses preferentially into the urine, causing a net secretion of anion from blood to urine. The concentrating power of the hippurate transport system is emphasized by the fact that secretion of the anion can, under certain experimental conditions, reverse the normal absorptive movement of water in S_2 segments to cause net fluid secretion. Organic anion secretion is inhibited competitively by probenecid.

The proximal tubule is heterogenous in respect to the number of organic anion transporters in the basolateral membrane of individual cells. The S_2 portions have more transporters per cell than the S_1 or S_3 segments; thus, more anion is secreted by the S_2 segment than by the S_1 and S_3 segments (Fig. 6-2).

Once the organic anions enter the urine, they generally flow through the remaining tubular segments without modification and without being actively reabsorbed. Some anionic drugs, however, may be absorbed by nonionic diffusion in the distal segments, in which case their elimination is strongly dependent on urinary pH (Chapter 5). Some amino acids are anionic at physiologic pH. These substances undergo secretion and reabsorption, but the mechanisms are poorly understood.

The organic anion system is especially important in clinical medicine. Many potent drugs and their metabolites are eliminated from the body in this way (Table 6-1). This tubular mechanism can also be used to

TABLE 6-1   ORGANIC MOLECULES SECRETED BY PROXIMAL TUBULES

Anions	Endogenous Compounds	Drugs
	Bile salts	Acetazolamide
	Cyclic AMP	Cephalothin
	Fatty acids	Chlorothiazide
	Hippurates	Ethacrynate
	Hydroxybenzoates	Furosemide
	Hydroxyindolacetate	Penicillin G
	Oxalate	Probenecid
	Prostaglandins	Saccharin
	Urate	Salicylate
Cations	Acetylcholine	Atropine
	Choline	Cimetidine
	Creatinine	Hexamethonium
	Dopamine	Morphine
	Epinephrine	Neostigmine
	Histamine	Paraquat
	Serotonin	Quinine
	Thiamine	Trimethoprim

assess renal function in patients. Radiolabelled hippurate (Hippuran) is used to evaluate patients with arterial hypertension and to assess the viability of nephrons in patients with acute and chronic renal failure. Since hippurate is taken up into proximal tubule cells from the blood side and concentrated in the cells by active transport, one can actually "see" evidence of living renal cells, even in patients who excrete no urine.

Figure 6-2 shows the appearance of the kidneys when viewed with a sensitive device that displays radioactive emissions on an oscilloscope. This example represents a patient with acute renal failure who was excreting no urine (anuria). One minute after the radioactive hippurate (Hippuran) was infused into an arm vein, the images of the kidneys were clearly seen. The images became even more intense as the hippurate accumulated in the tubule cells over several minutes. Thus the Hippuran image of the kidneys provides important information about renal viability even when no hippurate is excreted in the urine. The positive scan shows that (a) the blood vessels must be open in order for hippurate to enter the kidneys and (b) the proximal tubule cells must be alive, since the hippurate can only be accumulated by active transport.

The organic anion secretory mechanism does more than excrete metabolites. The system may be used to deliver biologically active substances from the proximal tubules to more distal sites. Prostaglandins are examples of endogenous substances and diuretics (furosemide and ethacrynic acid) are examples of exogenous chemicals that are delivered to sensitive distal sites after being secreted by the proximal tubules (Chapter 13 and Fig. 13-1).

Uric Acid

Approximately 8 to 12% of the filtered load of uric acid is excreted in the urine. Uric acid exists mainly as ionized urate in the plasma, and only in maximally acid urine is it in the undissociated acid form. The renal handling of urate is complex and different among animal species. In humans, urate is filtered freely, reabsorbed, and secreted as shown in Figure 6-3. Bidirectional transport (reabsorption and secretion) occurs exclusively in the proximal tubules. The relative strengths of the absorptive and secretory fluxes determines the net movement of urate, i.e., net secretion or net reabsorption, in each segment of the proximal tubule. It is thought that net urate reabsorption normally occurs in S_1 and S_3 segments and that net urate secretion occurs in S_2 segments. Normally, less urate leaves the proximal tubule in the tubular fluid than enters in the glomerular filtrate, that is, reabsorption predominates, so that the amount excreted in the urine is only 8 to 12% of that filtered. In some experimental settings, the clearance of urate can be made to exceed the clearance of inulin, indicating net secretion. This is due to an increased rate of urate secretion by the proximal tubules.

Urate absorption is inhibited by probenecid, and secretion is in-

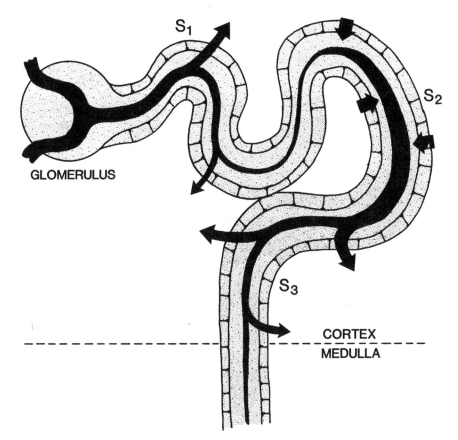

Figure 6-3. The proximal tubular absorption and secretion of urate.

hibited by pyrazinoic acid. Since pyrazinoic acid causes urate to nearly disappear from the urine, there is reason to believe that a great deal of the urate in the final urine derives from tubular secretion (Fig. 6-3).

Urate secretion is directly dependent on the plasma level of the anion. At high plasma levels, the excretion of urate increases strikingly due to increased tubular secretion. This powerful secretory process acts to keep the plasma urate levels within a normal range. Some patients with gout do not increase the renal secretion of urate normally when the endogenous production of urate is increased. These patients have high levels of urate in their plasma and frequently deposit urate crystals in joint fluid, causing gouty arthritis.

ORGANIC CATIONS

The function of the organic cation transport system is less well understood than that of the anion mechanisms. Some of the organic cations are bound to serum proteins and therefore are not filtered appreciably.

The cations are secreted by transporters located in the basolateral and luminal membranes of proximal tubular cells. N-methylnicotinamide (NMN) and tetraethylammonium (TEA) are prototypic cations, in the same way that PAH is representative of organic anion transport (Table 6-1).

Choline levels in the blood appear to be regulated by the renal organic cation transport system. Catecholamines and metabolites of these potent vasoactive agents are secreted into the urine by the organic cation system. Creatinine appears to be secreted to a small extent by this mechanism as well. In patients with moderate to advanced degrees of renal disease, this mechanism may account for a significant fraction of the creatinine excreted in the urine.

Clinically relevant drugs excreted by the organic cation system include atropine, morphine, quinine, trimethoprim, and cimetidine (Table 6-1). Since these substances compete for secretion by this system, one can inhibit the excretion of another and each can block the excretion of the endogenous organic cations as well. It is not uncommon to see an elevation of the serum creatinine level in patients receiving cimetidine or trimethoprim.

GLUCOSE, AMINO ACIDS, AND PLASMA PROTEINS

Several organic substances in plasma are filtered by the glomeruli, but normally do not appear in the urine in significant quantities because they are extensively reabsorbed by the renal tubules.

Glucose

D-glucose is a normal constituent of the plasma; approximately 750 mmoles are filtered each day. In normal adults, no glucose appears in the urine; therefore, the kidneys do not ordinarily regulate the plasma level of glucose. Most of the glucose is reabsorbed in the S_1 segment of the proximal tubule by a cotransport system tied to Na reabsorption (Chapter 7). The S_2 and S_3 portions can absorb the solute to a limited extent. In subjects with diabetes mellitus, the plasma glucose level rises far above the normal concentration of 5 mM, thereby increasing the quantity of glucose filtered by the glomeruli. When the plasma levels exceed about 15 mM, glucose is found in the urine since the quantity filtered exceeds the combined capacities of the proximal tubule segments to completely reabsorb it (Fig. 3-5).

Other sugars can be reabsorbed by the glucose transport mechanism in proximal tubules (i.e., D-galactose, D-fructose). There is no evidence to suggest that D-isomers are secreted into the urine.

Amino Acids

Many amino acids in the plasma are filtered by the glomeruli and are reabsorbed almost completely by the proximal tubules in cotransport with Na^+. Thus, the kidneys do not regulate the plasma levels of amino acids. The reabsorptive process favors the L- over the D-forms of the amino acids. Specific reabsorptive processes have been identified for neutral, diamino, and dicarboxylic amino acids; glycine; and beta amino acids. Cystine, and perhaps other amino acids, may be secreted into the urine under certain conditions.

Plasma Proteins

Small amounts of albumin (5 to 10 g per day) and much larger quantities of low molecular weight proteins and polypeptides leak through the glomerular membrane to appear in the tubule fluid. Yet, only about 50 to 150 mg/day of protein appears in the final urine in normal persons due to extensive reabsorption of these organic molecules by the proximal tubules.

Most of the proteins and polypeptides (including insulin, parathyroid hormone, angiotensin, and vasopressin) are absorbed by micropinocytotic processes in the apical membranes of proximal tubule cells. Most of these complex organic molecules are degraded inside the cells to smaller molecules, which in turn, are released through the basolateral plasma membrane to be recaptured by the peritubular capillaries.

Tamm-Horsfall protein is produced by cells in the thick ascending limbs and secreted into the urine. In highly concentrated, acidic, tubular fluid, the Tamm-Horsfall protein precipitates to form a cast in the tubule lumen. In certain disease states, this matrix material may entrap formed elements in tubule fluid (erythrocytes, leukocytes, tubule cells), which are excreted in the urine as cellular casts.

BIBLIOGRAPHY

General:

Chonko, A. M., and Grantham, J. J.: Disorders of Urate Metabolism and Excretion. *In* The Kidney. 2nd ed. Edited by B. M. Brenner, and F. C. Rector, Jr. Philadelphia, W. B. Saunders Co., 1981.

Irish, J. M. III, and Grantham, J. J.: Renal Handling of Organic Anions and Cations. *In* The Kidney. 2nd ed. Edited by B. M. Brenner, and F. C. Rector, Jr. Philadelphia, W. B. Saunders Co., 1981.

Rennick, B. R.: Renal tubule transport of organic cations. Am. J. Physiol., *240* (Renal Fluid Electrolyte Physiol. *9*): F83, 1981.

Schmidt-Nielsen, B.: Urea and the Kidney. Amsterdam, Excerpta Medica, 1970.

Specific:

Barfuss, D. W., and Schafer, J. A.: Active amino acid absorption by proximal convoluted and proximal straight tubules. Am. J. Physiol., *236* (Renal Fluid Electrolyte Physiol. *5*): F149, 1979.

Bourdeau, J. E. and Carone, F. A.: Protein handling by the renal tubule. Nephron, *13*:22, 1974.

Chonko, A. M.: Urate secretion in isolated rabbit renal tubules. Am. J. Physiol., *239* (Renal Fluid Electrolyte Physiol. *8*): F545, 1980.

Tune, B. M., and Burg, M. B.: Glucose transport by proximal renal tubules. Am. J. Physiol., *220*:87, 1971.

Tune, B. M., Burg, M. B., and Patlak, C. S.: Characteristics of p-aminohippurate transport in proximal renal tubules. Am. J. Physiol., *217*:1057, 1969.

CHAPTER 7
Mechanisms of Salt and Water Reabsorption

It is vitally important for the survival of an organism that both the osmotic concentration and the volume of its "internal environment," the extracellular fluid, be maintained constant. Since Na and its attendant anions are the major osmotic constituents of the extracellular fluid, the organism must control the amount of salt as well as the amount of water in this fluid. This is done primarily by controlling the rate of excretion of these substances; control of the intake of salt and water is usually, but not always, of secondary importance.

Within the kidney, the rate of excretion of salt and water is controlled by regulation of the GFR, described in Chapter 4, and by regulation of the rate of tubular reabsorption. To a great extent, water reabsorption occurs as a consequence of active salt reabsorption. Therefore, the primary tubular mechanisms involved in the maintenance of the osmotic concentration and volume of the extracellular fluid are the active transport systems for salt. The functioning of these systems and their influence on water reabsorption are affected by the anatomic structure of the various parts of the nephron, the activity of other transport systems within the nephron, and a variety of chemical and physical factors that arise from both inside and outside the kidney.

This complex subject is presented in the following way. In this chapter, the tubular mechanisms for salt and water reabsorption are described. In Chapter 8 we discuss how inhibition of specific tubular mechanisms result in increased excretion of salt and water, that is, diuresis. Finally, in Chapter 9, we discuss the reflex mechanisms that maintain the osmotic concentration and volume of the extracellular fluid by altering RBF, GFR, and tubular reabsorption.

PROXIMAL TUBULE

To recapitulate what has been stated in earlier chapters: The ultrafiltrate entering the proximal tubule has almost the same electrolyte and osmotic concentration as the plasma circulating in the capillaries that

119

surround the nephron. Some 60 to 70% of this fluid is normally reabsorbed and returned to the blood by the proximal tubule, with little change in Na or osmotic concentration of the remaining fluid (Fig. 5-5). The Cl concentration rises slightly and the HCO_3 concentration falls somewhat. This reabsorption is accomplished by an epithelial cell layer that has a high permeability to both water and small ions.

Several transport systems in the proximal tubule contribute to the reabsorption of salt and water, and there is a strong interdependence among them. In addition, the colloid osmotic pressure of the plasma in the peritubular capillaries surrounding the tubule contributes to the forces generating reabsorption.

Sodium Transport

The primary transport system driving salt and water reabsorption in the proximal tubule is the Na-K-ATPase mechanism residing in the basolateral membrane (see Chapter 1, Fig. 1-8). This mechanism pumps Na from the cell into the paracellular space and ISF and transports K in the opposite direction (Fig. 7-1). The reduction in cell Na concentration

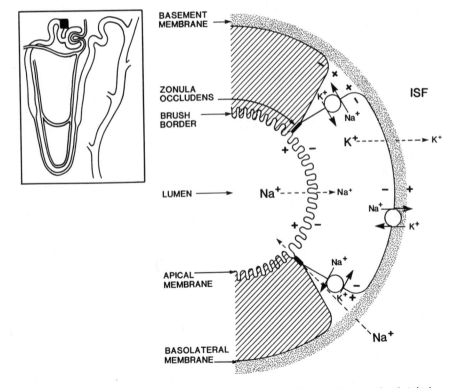

Figure 7-1. The mechanism for sodium reabsorption in the proximal tubule. ISF = interstitial fluid.

and rise in K concentration creates an electrochemical gradient favoring Na movement into the cell. The luminal membrane permits Na to enter the cell at a faster rate than does the basolateral membrane. Thus the combination of the pump in the basolateral membrane and the high Na permeability of the luminal membrane cause net Na movement in the reabsorptive direction. The active reabsorptive flux of Na tends to reduce the Na concentration in tubular fluid, establishing a transepithelial chemical gradient which can drive a passive back-flux through the paracellular pathway and into the tubular fluid. Because of the high permeability of this pathway to Na, the *net* rate of Na reabsorption is greatly limited by any factor that increases the gradient driving the passive back-flux.

In the early part of the proximal tubule, the entry of Na into the cell across the apical membrane is facilitated by a symport process that transports Na and glucose together. The cotransport is driven by the electrochemical gradient for Na across the apical membrane, which was established by the Na-K-ATPase system in the basolateral membrane. The symport molecular complex in the apical membrane will not transport either Na or glucose in the absence of the other. Similar symport systems exist for Na and various amino acids. Evidently, these symport processes exist also in later segments of the proximal tubule, but normally are not used because the tubular fluid concentration of glucose and amino acids fall to low levels in the early segments (Fig. 5-5).

Bicarbonate Reabsorption

Bicarbonate in the filtrate is reabsorbed by a complex process involving the secretion of hydrogen ions (Fig. 7-2). The apical membrane of proximal tubular cells secretes H ions from the cell into the tubular fluid. The secretion of the cation is electrically balanced by the movement of Na in the opposite direction. It is possible that this exchange occurs by an antiport system driven by the Na electrochemical gradient that exists across the apical membrane. Hydrogen ions entering the tubular fluid combine with HCO_3^- ions to form H_2O and CO_2. Thus the HCO_3^- ion disappears from the tubular fluid. In the cell, the fall in H^+ concentration drives the hydration of CO_2, which is catalyzed by the enzyme carbonic anhydrase. The HCO_3^- ion formed then moves out of the cell across the basolateral membrane by a transport process that is not understood. Thus the disappearance of a HCO_3^- ion from the tubular fluid is coupled to the appearance of another HCO_3^- ion in the interstitial fluid. The net result is the same as if a HCO_3^- ion were transported directly across the epithelium. Therefore the process is called bicarbonate reabsorption.

In the initial segment (S_1) of the proximal tubule, the fractional rate of HCO_3 reabsorption is faster than that for water, and the HCO_3 concentration of tubular fluid falls. As it falls, the H ion concentration rises (pH falls) and the rate of back-flux of H out of the tubule rises, decreasing the

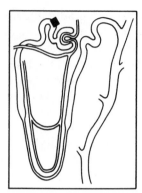
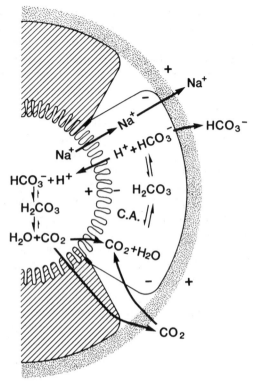

Figure 7-2. The mechanism for bicarbonate reabsorption in the proximal tubule. C. A. = carbonic anhydrase.

net secretion rate. Thus, at an early point along the tubule, the fractional rate of HCO_3 reabsorption declines to equal the rate of water reabsorption, and no further change in the tubular fluid concentration of HCO_3 occurs. This process is described in greater detail in Chapter 10.

Chloride Transport

Chloride reabsorption is driven primarily by electrochemical gradients established by active Na reabsorption. In the S_1 segment of the proximal tubule, the small transepithelial PD, lumen negative, may provide a driving force for Cl reabsorption via the paracellular pathway. However, the fractional rate of Cl reabsorption initially lags behind the rate of water reabsorption and the Cl concentration of tubular fluid increases to about 30% above the concentration in the interstitial fluid in the S_2 and S_3 segments. The rise in Cl concentration increases the electrochemical gradient for its reabsorption; the fractional rate of reabsorption rises to equal that of water reabsorption, and no further change in tubular fluid Cl concentration occurs until the fluid flows into the loop of Henle.

It is now recognized that a considerable amount of Cl may be reabsorbed through the cell as well as through the paracellular path. It is thought that a Na–Cl symport exists in the apical membrane which moves Na and Cl into the cell (Fig. 7-3). The transport process is driven by the electrochemical gradient for Na established by the Na-K-ATPase system. Little is known about the nature of the transport system that moves Cl out of the cell across the basolateral membrane.

Water Reabsorption

Water reabsorption occurs secondarily to the reabsorption of solute, chiefly NaCl. The removal of solute from the tubular fluid tends to reduce its osmotic concentration, and water passively flows across the epithelium into the ISF. Water moves so readily across the proximal tubular epithelium that whatever osmotic gradient exists across that wall is kept so small it cannot be measured. Until recently, it was difficult to understand how such a rapid rate of water movement could be generated by such a small osmotic gradient. Experimental work done on

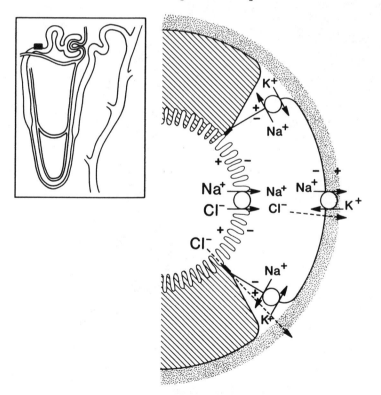

Figure 7-3. The mechanisms for chloride reabsorption in the proximal tubule. Chloride may be partially reabsorbed through the cell by a symport mechanism. It may also diffuse through the zonula occludens and the paracellular space in response to an electrochemical gradient.

other epithelial tissues, such as the rabbit gallbladder, the toad urinary bladder, and the gut of insects, suggests that movement of water across cell layers that transport solute may be facilitated by the presence in small intercellular spaces of a fluid with a somewhat higher osmotic concentration than exists in the fluid on both sides of the cell layer. This hypothesis, coupled with the discovery that the basolateral membrane surface area is much greater than was previously realized, has led to the current theory on the mechanism of fluid reabsorption from the proximal tubule.

The labyrinth of intercellular channels formed by interdigitating, cytoplasmic lamellae was described in Chapter 5 (Figs. 5-1, 5-2). These channels open onto the permeable basement membrane and are closed off from the lumen by the less permeable zonula occludens. According to the current hypothesis, the cell membranes lining these channels transport solute, chiefly Na, Cl, and HCO_3, into the fluid within the channels, making that fluid slightly hyperosmotic (Fig. 7-4). The appli-

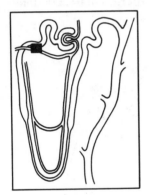
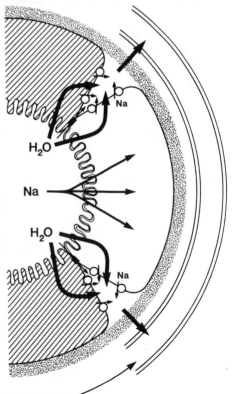

PERITUBULAR CAPILLARY

Figure 7-4. Water reabsorption in the proximal tubule. The transport of Na and other solutes into the paracellular space establishes a small osmotic gradient that drives H_2O into the paracellular space.

cation of that small osmotic force to a large membrane surface area induces a flow of water from the cell and thence from the lumen into the channels. The accumulation of fluid within the channels raises the hydrostatic pressure, which causes a bulk flow of water and solute across the permeable basement membrane at the open end of the channel.

The osmotic concentration of the paracellular fluid may be only 2 to 3 mOsm/kg H_2O higher than the concentration of the tubular fluid and the plasma in the peritubular capillaries. That is, however, equivalent to 39 to 58 mm Hg. The reabsorption of that hyperosmotic fluid from the tubule would reduce the osmotic concentration of tubular fluid, but the expected fall in concentration (< 5 mOsm/kg H_2O or 1/60 of the total concentration) is less than the error of currently available techniques for measuring the osmotic concentration of small tubular fluid samples.

The reabsorbed fluid leaving the intercellular channels must enter the peritubular capillaries in order to return to the circulation. Fluid movement into the capillaries is governed by the balance of the hydrostatic and oncotic pressures of the capillary (Fig. 7-5). The oncotic pressure of the peritubular capillary plasma (π_b) is higher than that of plasma elsewhere in the body because of the loss of protein-free fluid by filtration at the glomerulus (see Fig. 4-1). The magnitude of the rise in π_b varies with the fraction of the renal plasma flow that is filtered (filtration fraction = GFR/RPF). The peritubular capillary hydrostatic pressure (P_{pc}) is controlled to a great extent by the degree of constriction of the efferent arteriole upstream. An increase in constriction reduces P_{pc}. This pressure may also be influenced by the hematocrit of the blood leaving the glomerulus. An increase in hematocrit tends to increase blood viscosity, which causes the resistance to blood flow in the efferent arterioles to rise; this, in turn, causes P_{pc} to fall. The hematocrit of the blood in the efferent arterioles is high because of the loss of cell-free fluid in the glomerulus, and it varies with changes in the filtration fraction in the same manner as does π_b. The net effect of these factors is to maintain π_b high and P_{pc} low, so that the net force for reabsorption is high.

If the filtration fraction falls or if efferent arteriolar constriction is reduced, the rate of movement of fluid from the paracellular space into the capillary is reduced. Presumably, this would cause the hydrostatic pressure in the paracellular labyrinth to rise. This would slow the rate of fluid reabsorption from the tubule, although how this may occur is not fully understood. One strong possibility is that a rise in pressure within the labyrinth may increase the back-flux of water and solute into the tubule through the zonula occludens. Evidence suggests that the flux of solute through the zonula occludens does increase during the diuresis that results from a large intake of salt and water.

Net hydrostatic and oncotic pressure differences exist between the

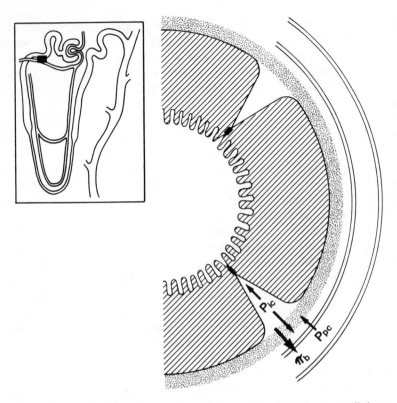

Figure 7-5. The pressures involved in fluid movement from the paracellular space into the capillaries. P_{ic} = hydrostatic pressure in the intercellular space. π_b = colloid osmotic pressure of plasma in the peritubular capillary. P_{pc} = hydrostatic pressure in the peritubular capillary.

tubular lumen and the peritubular capillary. The hydrostatic pressure of the tubular fluid is higher than that of the capillary plasma; the colloid osmotic pressure is much lower. It must be emphasized, however, that these gradients do not directly cause fluid movement out of the tubule. Fluid leaves the tubule and enters the paracellular labyrinth only under the influence of the osmotic gradient created primarily by the active transport of Na. The hydrostatic and colloid osmotic pressure gradients are considered to affect fluid movement only from that point on into the capillary.

To summarize both the known facts and the current hypothesis in regard to water reabsorption from the proximal tubule: the active transport of solute, chiefly salt, into the paracellular labyrinth raises the osmotic pressure of the fluid in that space slightly above that in the cell and tubular lumen. That small osmotic force applied to a large membrane surface area causes the flow of water into the paracellular space. This raises the hydrostatic pressure in that space, which causes a bulk flow of water and solute across the basement membrane. The high colloid osmotic pressure in the peritubular capillaries causes absorption of that fluid into the capillaries. The reabsorbed fluid leaving the tubule may be slightly hyperosmotic; thus, the remaining tubular fluid may become slightly hypo-osmotic.

Summary

Salt and water reabsorption from the proximal tubule is primarily generated by active transport of Na from the cell across the basolateral membrane. The electrochemical gradients established by the Na-K-ATPase system drive Cl reabsorption. The small osmotic force generated by salt transport causes the reabsorption of water, which is facilitated by the high colloid osmotic pressure of plasma in the peritubular capillary. The secretion of H ions contributes to the reabsorption of Na and water by causing the reabsorption of bicarbonate.

Na transport is the main active and primary event. The transport of Cl and water is passive and secondary to the active transport of Na. Because of the high conductance and high water permeability of the epithelium, all these transport processes are highly interdependent. Any small interference in the reabsorption of any solute, or in the reabsorption of water, affects the reabsorption of all the others. For instance, inhibition of Na reabsorption will obviously inhibit transport of Cl and water. Any interference with water reabsorption will slow Na and Cl reabsorption, since solute reabsorption without water reabsorption would begin to drop the solute concentration in tubular fluid. The resulting transepithelial chemical gradient would increase the back-flux of solute into the nephron and reduce the net rate of solute transport. Water reabsorption can be slowed by the accumulation of impermeant, poorly reabsorbed solute in the tubular fluid. This accumulation would oppose the osmotic force causing water reabsorption.

The net result of the work of these interdependent transport mechanisms is the bulk reabsorption of 60 to 70% of the filtrate with only minor changes in the osmotic and electrolyte concentrations of the tubular fluid flowing into the loop of Henle.

LOOP OF HENLE

The descending segment of the thin limb possesses no known active transport systems, but it is highly permeable to water. Water reabsorption can occur if an osmotic gradient exists between the tubular fluid and the surrounding interstitial fluid. In the cortex, the interstitial fluid has an osmotic concentration close to that of the tubular fluid, so it is probable that little reabsorption occurs in the thin limb of superficial cortical nephrons. However, the environment of the thin limb of juxtamedullary nephrons is different. The concentrations of Na, Cl, and urea in the medullary interstitial fluid progressively increase at each level from the corticomedullary junction to the tip of the papilla. Thus, as tubular fluid in the thin limb flows down into the medulla, it is exposed to an ever-increasing osmotic concentration in the interstitial fluid surrounding the permeable epithelium. Water reabsorption in response to that gradient causes the tubular fluid osmotic concentration to progressively increase as it flows toward the tip of the loop.

Solute entry into the tubular fluid from the concentrated medullary ISF could also occur if the epithelium were permeable to solutes. This is a controversial question. Direct in vitro measurements on the thin descending limb of the rabbit indicate that the epithelium has a low permeability to Na and urea. Indirect in vivo measurements in other species strongly indicate that significant solute entry does occur.

In superficial cortical nephrons, the thin limb ends before the tip of the loop of Henle is reached (Fig. 2-2). In juxtamedullary nephrons, however, there is a long ascending segment of the thin limb. Despite the absence of gross morphologic differences, the functional properties of the ascending segment differ considerably from those of the descending segment. The water permeability of the ascending segment is low and there is movement of solute out of the tubular fluid. Thus, the tubular fluid becomes hypotonic to the surrounding medullary ISF.

The mechanism of transport of solute has not been definitively established. Active transport of Na has been proposed to occur here, but the evidence is not convincing. Another theory is based on the finding that the permeability of the ascending thin limb of the rabbit to Na is higher than its permeability to urea. It is proposed that the Na concentration of tubular fluid in the thin ascending limb is higher than in the medullary ISF and that a gradient for urea exists in the opposite direction. According to the theory, the relative permeabilities and concentration gradients for NaCl and urea permit NaCl to diffuse out of the lumen faster than urea can enter. The net loss of solute dilutes the tubular fluid. However, the existence of the requisite concentration gradients has not been established.

The process of dilution of the tubular fluid by reabsorption of solute continues as the tubular fluid flows through the thick ascending limb, and the tubular fluid osmotic concentration may be 150 to 200 mOsm/kg H_2O less than the osmotic concentration of the surrounding interstitium. The mechanism of dilution of the tubular fluid by the thick limb has been more thoroughly studied than that in the thin ascending limb. It is apparent that active solute transport occurs across an epithelium with a low permeability to water and a relatively low conductance to small ions.

The nature of the active solute transport system in the thick limb has been in doubt. Initially, it was postulated that Na was actively reabsorbed. Later, it was discovered that the transepithelial electrical potential difference was 4 to 10 mV, lumen positive, indicating that Cl was being absorbed against a steeper electrochemical gradient than Na. This led to the hypothesis that active Cl reabsorption generated the electrical gradient and that Na reabsorption was secondary to Cl reabsorption. This was reinforced by the observation that the transepithelial PD fell towards zero when Cl was replaced by nitrate. This hypothesis does not explain the finding that ouabain, which inhibits Na-K-ATPase, blocked Cl reabsorption. Since it is known that Na-K-ATPase exists in high concentration in the basolateral membrane of thick ascending limb cells, it now seems more probable that active Na transport out of the cell across the basolateral membrane is the primary active process. Both Na and Cl may move from the lumen into the cell by a cotransport or symport process existing within the apical membrane. This entry process presumably is driven by the electrochemical gradient for Na established by Na-K-ATPase. Explanation of the transepithelial PD requires a more thorough knowledge of the properties of the apical and basolateral membranes and the paracellular pathway than presently exists.

The relatively low Na and Cl conductances of the epithelium reduce back-flux of these ions from the interstitium into the tubular fluid. This, coupled with the low water permeability of the epithelium, enables the transport mechanisms to reduce the Na and Cl concentrations in tubular fluid to less than 50% of those in the surrounding interstitium.

The low water permeability of the epithelium does not permit significant water reabsorption to accompany solute reabsorption. Reabsorption of salt without water continually dilutes the tubular fluid so that the osmotic concentration falls to about 150 mOsm/kg H_2O in tubular fluid flowing into the distal tubule. It is important to remember that this also results in more salt than water being transported into the medullary interstitial fluid by the entire loop of Henle, thereby causing the osmotic concentration of the ISF to rise.

The loop of Henle reabsorbs 15 to 20% of the filtrate and passes 20 to 30% on to the distal tubule. The fraction of the filtered NaCl reabsorbed is greater than the fraction of filtered water reabsorbed (Fig. 5-6).

DISTAL TUBULE

The distal convoluted tubule is a heterogeneous unit of the nephron both in structure (see Chapter 5) and in function. The initial segment functions much as an extension of the thick ascending limb. Its permeability to water is low and active salt transport continues to dilute the tubular fluid. The more distal segments of the tubule may function differently. In some species at least, this segment is sensitive to antidiuretic hormone (ADH), and in its presence, becomes permeable to water. Moreover, transport and electrical properties of the distal segment combine to create a large transepithelial potential difference of 40 to 50 mV, lumen negative.

In the absence of antidiuretic hormone, the entire tubule acts as a diluting segment. The permeability to water is low throughout its length, and active salt reabsorption continues to dilute the hypotonic tubular fluid arriving from the loop of Henle. Some water is reabsorbed so the volume delivered to the collecting tubule is reduced, but active salt reabsorption further reduces the osmotic concentration to approximately 80 to 100 mOsm/kg H_2O.

In the presence of antidiuretic hormone, the osmotic concentration of the cortical interstitial fluid (285 mOsm/kg H_2O) drives water reabsorption across the permeable late segments, and the osmotic concentration of the tubular fluid rises to the isosmotic level. In this situation, 5 to 8% of the glomerular filtrate is reabsorbed by the distal tubule.

The permeability or conductance of the distal tubular epithelium to Na is lower than in more proximal segments of the nephron. Thus, active reabsorption of Na can reduce the tubular fluid concentration to about 25% of the plasma concentration before the rate of passive backflux becomes sufficient to prevent further reabsorption. The mineralocorticoid hormones stimulate Na reabsorption in the distal tubule, and in their absence, the ability of the epithelium to reduce the tubular fluid Na concentration to low levels is compromised.

Chloride is also reabsorbed against an electrochemical gradient. It is probable that reabsorption occurs by a cotransport system similar to that described for the thick ascending limb. Bicarbonate reabsorption again occurs as a result of hydrogen secretion. Since the epithelium can establish a larger transepithelial hydrogen concentration gradient than is possible in the proximal tubule, the bicarbonate concentration of tubular fluid can be reduced to much lower levels.

The amounts of water, sodium, chloride, and bicarbonate reabsorbed by the distal tubule are much less than the amounts reabsorbed by the proximal tubule. In addition, the low permeability of the epithelium to electrolytes and the influence of ADH and mineralocorticoid hormones reduce the close interdependence of solute and water reabsorption that is seen in the proximal tubule. Because of this, the osmotic and Na, Cl, and HCO_3 concentrations can vary over much wider ranges.

COLLECTING TUBULE

The epithelium of the collecting tubule throughout its length is a "tight" epithelium in terms of its permeability to electrolytes, its electrical resistance, and in the absence of ADH, its permeability to water. When ADH secretion is reduced to low levels, the hypotonic fluid entering the collecting tubule is further diluted by active salt reabsorption to an osmotic concentration as low as 40 to 60 mOsm/kg H_2O. This low concentration can be achieved even though the osmotic concentration of the medullary interstitial fluid surrounding the tubule may be higher than 600 mOsm/kg H_2O. Little water is reabsorbed along the entire length of the collecting tubule, and as much as 20 L/day, 11% of the filtered water, may be excreted.

When ADH secretion is stimulated, the tubular fluid flowing from the distal tubule into the collecting tubule is nearly isosmotic with the cortical interstitial fluid. ADH causes the luminal membranes of collecting tubular cells to be highly permeable to water. In the cortical sections of the tubule, active salt reabsorption tends to create an osmotic gradient and water is then easily reabsorbed in response to small osmotic forces. The result is that a small volume of isosmotic tubular fluid flows into the medullary sections of the collecting tubule. There the high osmotic concentration of the medullary interstitial fluid, created by active salt reabsorption from the loop of Henle, is able to exert its influence and water is reabsorbed from the duct, gradually raising the osmotic concentration of the tubular fluid as it flows toward the papillary tip. The final osmotic concentration of the urine may approach 1400 mOsm/kg H_2O in the human, and the volume excreted may be as low as 0.3% of the filtrate.

The volumes of water reabsorbed by the cortical and medullary sections of the nephron are different when ADH is present. The medullary collecting tubules serve to concentrate the urine to the maximal extent by reabsorbing about 5% of the filtered water. By contrast, the cortical sections may remove about 15% of the filtered water. The clinical importance of these factors is seen in patients who have diseases that cause destruction of the papillae (papillary necrosis). The patients can dilute the urine to osmolalities below that of plasma and they respond to ADH by increasing urine osmolality to the same level as plasma. In this way, some degree of regulation of water balance can be maintained even though the papillae may be absent.

The electrical resistance of the paracellular pathway in the collecting tubule is greater and the conductance to small ions is smaller than in the rest of the nephron. The transepithelial potential difference varies widely along the length of the tubule; it may also vary widely with time in any one segment.

Na is actively reabsorbed by the collecting tubular epithelium at lower rates than in the rest of the nephron. The low conductance of the paracellular pathway permits only small rates of back-flux, so the concentration of Na in tubular fluid can be reduced to less than 1 mM. As in the distal tubule, Na reabsorption is stimulated by mineralocortoids. Cl is reabsorbed against an electrochemical gradient by an unknown mechanism. Its concentration in tubular fluid can also be reduced to low levels. Hydrogen ion secretion is capable of reducing the tubular fluid pH to less than 4.5. At this level, the bicarbonate concentration of tubular fluid would be very low (< 0.1 mM).

Because of the extreme variations that can occur in water reabsorption by the collecting tubular epithelium, the concentration of salt in the urine leaving the kidney varies from less than 1 mM to more than twice the plasma concentration. This variability is compounded by the action of the mineralocorticoids on salt reabsorption. The ability to vary *almost* independently the volume of water and the amount of salt transported by the collecting tubule assists the organism in maintaining homeostasis of the volume and composition of the extracellular fluid in the face of changes in intake of salt and water.

SUMMARY

The salt reabsorptive mechanisms are the primary transport processes involved in the control of the volume and osmotic concentration of the extracellular fluid. Throughout the nephron, they serve to generate the osmotic gradients that bring about the passive and secondary reabsorption of water. The largest bulk of the filtrate is reabsorbed in the proximal tubule. Here, the volume reabsorbed can be altered by a variety of factors, but the osmotic concentration never varies from that of the plasma. In the more distal structures, the variable permeability of the tubular epithelium to water, the low permeability to electrolytes, and the variable rates of salt transport permit reabsorption of salt and water in varying proportions so that the electrolyte and osmotic concentrations as well as the volume of urine can fluctuate over a wide range.

THE DILUTION PROCESS

When water intake is excessive and ADH secretion is suppressed, the kidney is able to excrete copious amounts of water without a large increase in solute excretion. This permits the organism to maintain the osmotic concentration of the extracellular fluid constant without large changes in its volume.

The kidney dilutes the urine and increases water excretion by reabsorption of solute in the distal segments of the nephron, as described earlier, when the absence of ADH has reduced the permeability of the tubular epithelium to water. The thick ascending limb and the initial section of the distal convoluted tubule are often called the diluting segment because it is in this segment that fractional reabsorption of solute always exceeds fractional water reabsorption whether ADH is absent or not. It is in this segment that the osmotic concentration of the tubular fluid falls below that of the glomerular filtrate. If ADH is absent, fractional solute reabsorption continues to exceed fractional water reabsorption in succeeding segments of the nephron. In the human, water excretion can reach as high as 20 L or 11% of the GFR per day. The osmotic concentration of this urine can be as low as 40 to 60 mOsm/kg H_2O.

The kidney also has the ability to do the opposite: to increase fractional water reabsorption so that it exceeds fractional solute reabsorption. The urine volume can be reduced to less than 1 L per day and the solute concentration may approach 1400 mOsm/kg H_2O. The concentration process is much more complex and involves much more than increased secretion of ADH and a high permeability of the tubular epithelium to water.

THE CONCENTRATION PROCESS: COUNTERCURRENT MECHANISM

The mechanism the kidney uses to osmotically concentrate the urine involves all the tubular structures and the capillaries in the medulla. They interact with each other and the medullary interstitial fluid so as to produce and conserve a unique hyperosmotic environment within the medulla. Basically, the osmotic gradient, created across the epithelium of the thick ascending limb by active transport of salt without the concomitant reabsorption of water, is conserved and multiplied by the countercurrent flow of urine in the loop of Henle and of blood in the medullary capillaries, the vasa recta. This countercurrent osmotic gradient then drives water reabsorption from the collecting tubule.

The Countercurrent Principle

There are many examples of the use of the countercurrent principle in biologic systems. However, the principle was usefully applied by engineers long before biologists became aware of its existence. Indeed, the possibility that the countercurrent principle is used by the kidney was suggested by physical chemists.

The countercurrent principle is most easily illustrated by considering a furnace (Fig. 7-6) in which the fresh air duct lies side by side with the exhaust duct so that fresh air entering the furnace flows counter to and in close proximity with the exhaust fumes. The cold air flowing into the furnace receives heat from the exhaust fumes, and a small horizontal temperature gradient between the two pipes is "multiplied" into a large vertical gradient. The air entering the furnace arrives at a high temperature and the heat that could have been lost in the exhaust is conserved, thereby improving the efficiency of the furnace.

Application to the Kidney

It was first noticed that the hairpin construction of the loops of Henle and the vasa recta form ideal countercurrent flow patterns which conceivably could participate in the osmotic concentration of the urine. Investigations made with this hypothesis in mind produced the following observations. The solute content of medullary tissue was found to progressively increase in serial sections beginning near the cortex and reaching toward the papilla. Tubular fluid also becomes progressively more concentrated as it flows down the collecting tubule through the medulla. In the tip of the papilla, where the urine in the collecting duct

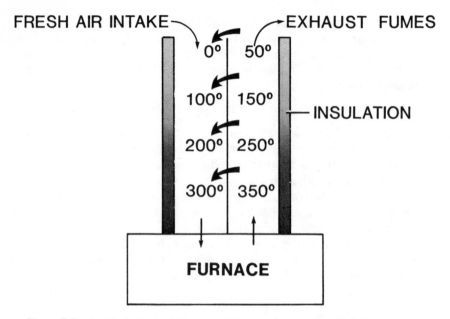

Figure 7-6. An illustration of the use of the countercurrent principle to conserve heat and improve the efficiency of a furnace. The thick arrows indicate the direction of heat flow.

is most concentrated, the fluid within the tip of the loop of Henle and the blood in the vasa recta are as highly concentrated as the urine. Finally, fluid in the beginning of the distal tubule was discovered to be hypo-osmotic to its surroundings and to have a low Na and Cl concentration. This indicated, first, that an active reabsorptive mechanism for NaCl probably exists in the ascending limb and, second, that the ascending limb has a low permeability to water. This discovery suggested that active solute transport provides the key generating force (the furnace) that is "multiplied" and conserved by the countercurrent flows in the loops of Henle and the vasa recta.

These observations and others can be summed up as follows: a gradient of osmotic concentration down the length of the medulla ranges from 285 mOsm/kg H_2O near the cortex to 1500 to 5000 mOsm/kg H_2O (depending on the particular species) in the papilla. This gradient exists in the interstitial fluid (ISF), in the urine within the loops of Henle, and in the blood within the vasa recta. When the animal is in the nondiuretic state, at any one level in the medulla, the interstitial fluid, the blood in the vasa recta, the urine in the descending limb of the loop of Henle and in the collecting tubule have approximately the same osmotic concentration. The urine within the ascending limb has a somewhat lower concentration, which is caused by the removal of more salt than water by the tubular epithelium. These findings and studies of the characteristics of the structures involved have led to a fuller, but still incomplete, understanding of the complex process by which the urine is osmotically concentrated.

Anatomy and Characteristics of the Structures Involved

The countercurrent system works within the confines of the medulla of the kidney. The anatomy of the medulla is illustrated in Figure 2-1. The important anatomic feature is the long hairpin construction of the loops of Henle and the vasa recta, which provide the "countercurrents." In these structures, the tubular fluid and blood flowing up and out of the medulla run counter to and in close proximity with tubular fluid and blood flowing down into the medulla. The collecting tubules bring a smaller volume of the tubular fluid from the cortex through the medulla, through the hypertonic environment established and preserved by the hairpin countercurrent loops.

The following characteristics of the medullary structures are of special importance to the countercurrent mechanism. The descending limbs of the loop are highly permeable to water. The degree of their permeability to Na, Cl, and urea is controversial. No active transepithelial transport of solute is known to occur in this structure. The ascending limb actively reabsorbs Na and Cl and is relatively impermeable to water. The vasa recta are considered to be highly permeable to Na, Cl, urea, and water. Some evidence, however, suggests that these capillaries may be different from others and it is possible that the descending and ascending sections may differ from each other. The collecting tubules are relatively impermeable to Na and Cl; their permeability to water is controlled by ADH. Cortical and outer medullary segments of the collecting tubule are poorly permeable to urea, but the inner medullary segment is permeable.

All the tubular structures and the vasa recta interact with each other through the medium in which they are bathed, the medullary interstitial fluid. Each structure tends to alter the composition of that fluid, and in turn, that fluid influences solute and water movement across the wall of each structure. The medullary interstitial fluid is not well mixed. Remember that the time required for diffusion of a solute within a fluid increases as a function of the square of the increase in distance over which exchange must occur. Thus, the progressively increasing solute concentration in that fluid from the cortico–medullary junction to the papilla can be preserved by the countercurrent mechanism acting upon solute and water transport across small horizontal distances, despite diffusion along the relatively large vertical length of the medulla.

"Countercurrent Multiplier": The Loop of Henle

The primary generating force for the countercurrent system is the active transport mechanism for salt in the ascending limb of the loop of Henle (Fig. 7-7). It removes solute from the tubular fluid and deposits

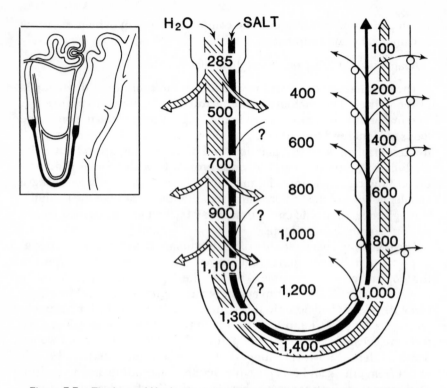

Figure 7-7. The loop of Henle, the "countercurrent multiplier." The numbers indicate the osmotic concentration in mOsm/kg H_2O of the tubular fluid and the interstitial fluid. The active transport of salt without water out of the ascending limb increases the osmotic concentration of the medullary interstitium. The small horizontal gradient is multiplied vertically by countercurrent flow. Water is reabsorbed from the descending limb by this osmotic force. Note that tubular fluid flows out of the loop at an osmotic concentration lower than that of the entering fluid. Fractionally more solute than water has been lost to the medullary interstitium.

it in the medullary ISF. The impermeability of the tubular wall slows the rate at which water follows solute out, so the osmotic concentration of the tubular fluid is reduced and the concentration of the ISF is raised. It is this initial small, horizontal osmotic gradient across the tubular wall that is "multiplied" vertically along the length of the loop by countercurrent flow.

The hyperosmotic concentration of the ISF then causes water to move out of the descending limb, thereby progressively raising the concentration of the remaining tubular fluid as it flows toward the tip of the loop. Na and Cl may diffuse from the medullary ISF back into the tubular fluid in the descending limb. This also serves to increase its osmotic concentration. After the fluid flows around the bend and starts back up in the ascending limb, Na and Cl, but little water, are removed and the fluid becomes more and more dilute as it approaches the distal tubule.

It is important to realize that fluid enters the medulla in the descending limb with an osmotic concentration of 285 mOsm/kg H_2O and leaves the medulla in the ascending limb with an osmotic concentration of approximately 100 mOsm/kg H_2O. Fractionally more solute than water is removed from the tubular fluid by the loop. Some of this excess solute is deposited in the medullary ISF, raising its osmotic concentration. This creates the osmotic force that causes water to move out of the other structures in the medulla.

Of course, the osmotic concentration of the medulla does not rise *ad infinitum* as the loop of Henle continues to deposit solute there. Some of this reabsorbed solute is carried away by the blood flow in the vasa recta. The amount of solute leaving the medulla via this route must increase as the osmotic concentration of the medulla increases, until a steady state is reached in which the amount of solute leaving the tubular fluid equals the amount carried away by the vasa recta.

Roles of the Distal Tubule and Collecting Duct

The distal tubules in the cortex receive the hypo-osmotic tubular fluid from the loop of Henle and reduce its volume by reabsorption of solute and water (Fig. 7-8). In the presence of ADH, the cortical sections of the collecting tubules permit the tubular fluid to lose water so that it comes into osmotic equilibrium with the cortical ISF. They also reabsorb additional solute and water. Thus, the solute-free water, formed by salt reabsorption in the ascending limb, is returned to the systemic circulation not to the medullary interstitial fluid, and a much smaller volume of isosmotic, tubular fluid reenters the medulla. As the tubular fluid comes into contact with the hyperosmotic environment of the medulla, water flows out into the interstitial space and the remaining urine becomes increasingly more concentrated as it approaches the papilla.

The water leaving the collecting tubule and entering the medullary ISF tends to dilute the solute in that fluid. However, the amount of solute pumped into the interstitial space by the loop of Henle is proportionately greater. This is because the hypo-osmotic tubular fluid leaving the loop of Henle loses water in the cortex before it reenters the medulla. The greater the ratio of solute to water reabsorbed from the medullary structures, the greater will be the osmotic concentration of the medullary interstitial fluid, resulting in a higher osmotic concentration of the final urine.

"Countercurrent Exchanger": The Vasa Recta

If the blood vessels in the medulla were anatomically similar to those in the cortex, it would be difficult for the loop of Henle to maintain the countercurrent osmotic gradient. However, the hairpin construction of the vasa recta, coupled with a blood flow rate that is much slower than the flow rate in the cortex, allows blood to flow through medullary tissue

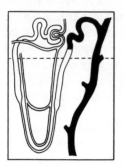
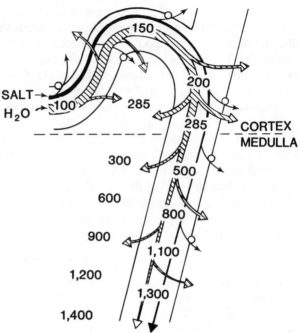

Figure 7-8. The role of the distal tubule and collecting duct in the countercurrent process. Hypo-osmotic fluid received from the loop of Henle loses water and solute to the *cortical* interstitium and a much smaller volume of isosmotic fluid flows into the medullary collecting tubule. Here water is reabsorbed into the hyperosmotic medullary interstitium, raising the osmotic concentration of the urine.

without causing more than a minimal disturbance in the osmotic gradient.

Plasma enters the descending limb of the vasa recta with the usual systemic osmotic concentration of 285 mOsm/kg H_2O (Fig. 7-9). As it flows down through the medulla, it comes into contact through the capillary wall with the high Na, Cl, and osmotic concentration of the medullary ISF. Water flows out of the descending limb as a result of the osmotic gradient, and Na and Cl diffuse in. Thus, the plasma becomes increasingly more concentrated as it approaches the tip of the papilla. As this concentrated fluid flows into the ascending limb of the vasa recta and back towards the cortex, it encounters interstitial fluid that is more dilute than it is. Water then flows down the osmotic gradient into the ascending vasa recta and Na and Cl diffuse out as a result of the concentration gradient.

The net result of this countercurrent flow into and out of the hyperosmotic medullary environment is the preservation of the high solute concentration of the medulla. Excess water is kept out of the medulla because it tends to "short circuit" the loop by leaving the dilute incoming plasma and flowing into the more concentrated plasma leaving the medulla. In addition, most of the solute deposited in the medulla by the loop of Henle is kept trapped there because it diffuses into the dilute plasma entering the medulla and back out again from the concentrated plasma leaving the medulla.

It is apparent that, despite the efficiency of the countercurrent exchange, the vasa recta carries away more solute from the medulla than it brings. It also carries away water reabsorbed from the collecting duct. Since proportionately more solute than water is reabsorbed by the tubu-

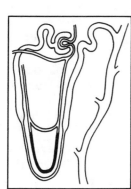
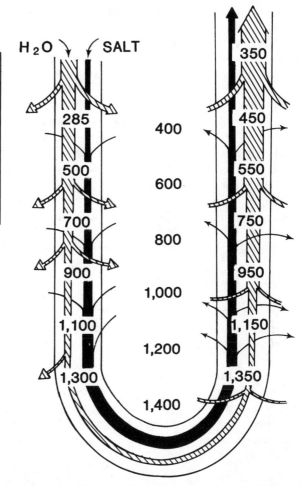

Figure 7-9. The vasa recta, the "countercurrent exchanger." Isosmotic plasma flowing into the medulla loses water to and gains solute from the medullary interstitium. As the hyperosmotic blood flows up the ascending limb, the process is reversed. However, there is a net gain of both water and solute. The exiting plasma flow is greater than that entering and is slightly hyperosmotic.

lar structures in the medulla, the plasma leaving the medulla must be hyperosmotic.

The colloid osmotic pressure of the plasma probably causes the net movement of fluid from the interstitial space into the ascending vasa recta. That pressure exceeds the hydrostatic pressure, which is quite low, partially because of the high resistance to flow in these long capillaries.

The Role of Urea

This description of the countercurrent mechanism has thus far focused on the transport of Na and Cl and the effect of that transport on water reabsorption. Indeed, it is the active transport of NaCl out of the ascending thick limb that is the primary generating force for the countercurrent mechanism. Urea also plays a major role in the osmotic concentration of the urine. The countercurrent system can concentrate urea in the tubular fluid and thus increase the total solute concentration of the urine. Experiments have also shown that a reduction in the supply of urea to the kidney reduces the effectiveness of the countercurrent trapping of NaCl in the medullary interstitial fluid and decreases the concentration of nonurea solute in the final urine. However, a full understanding of the role of urea has proved elusive.

The means by which urea itself is concentrated in the medullary interstitial fluid is fairly straightforward. About 40% of the filtered urea is reabsorbed in the proximal tubule, and because water is reabsorbed to a greater extent, the urea concentration in tubular fluid rises about 50% (Fig. 5-5). Somewhere between the end of the convoluted tubule and the tip of the loop of Henle, urea is added to the tubular fluid; as a result, the concentration in tubular fluid at the tip is high. Urea may be added by active secretion in the straight segment of the proximal tubule or by passive diffusion from the medullary interstitial fluid into the descending limb of the loop of Henle. From the tip of the loop through the ascending limb, the distal tubule, and the cortical and outer medullary sections of the collecting tubule, the concentration of urea in tubular fluid continues to rise as the rate of water reabsorption exceeds the rate of urea reabsorption (Figs. 5-5 and 7-10). As a consequence, the concentration of urea in tubular fluid reaching the inner medullary segment of the collecting tubule is high. This segment of the nephron is permeable to urea and it diffuses readily into the medullary interstitial fluid, raising its urea concentration (Fig. 7-10). From there urea diffuses into the blood flowing through the vasa recta. Blood flowing up the ascending vasa recta and out of the inner medulla carries urea at a high concentration into the outer medulla, where it diffuses out into the interstitial space and also into the blood flowing down into the medulla. By this process, urea reabsorbed into the medullary ISF from the collect-

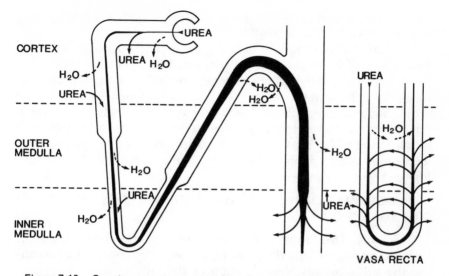

Figure 7-10. Countercurrent concentration of urea by the vasa recta and collecting ducts. Urea reabsorption occurs at a slower rate than water reabsorption throughout most of the nephron, so its concentration in tubular fluid rises. In the inner medullary sections of the collecting tubule, the high concentration in tubular fluid drives passive diffusion into the medullary interstitium. Here urea is trapped by the countercurrent flow of the vasa recta, which raises the concentration in the medullary interstitium.

ing duct is trapped and recycled by the vasa recta and the urea concentration in the medullary ISF climbs to a high level.

One current theory on the role of urea in the countercurrent mechanism suggests the following: The addition of urea to the medullary ISF raises the osmotic force acting to withdraw water from the descending limb of the loop, which is considered to be poorly permeable to Na and Cl. This raises the Na and Cl concentrations in tubular fluid reaching the tip of the loop above that in the surrounding ISF. As the fluid flows into the thin ascending limb, a gradient exists for Na and Cl diffusion out across an epithelium permeable to the ions but not to water. The loss of Na and Cl reduces the osmotic concentration of tubular fluid and raises the osmotic concentration of the ISF. If the countercurrent trapping of urea is reduced, the gradient for Na and Cl diffusion out of the ascending limb is reduced and the trapping of NaCl in the medullary ISF is slowed. Acceptance of this theory requires unequivocal demonstration, first, that a NaCl concentration gradient exists between thin ascending limb fluid and the medullary ISF that is sufficient to account for the dilution of tubular fluid that takes place and, second, that this gradient is dependent on urea trapping.

Another theory is based on the fact that the papilla of the kidney protrudes into the renal pelvis and is bathed by the urine exiting from the collecting ducts. This theory suggests that urea diffusion from the highly concentrated urine into the medullary ISF contributes to the total osmotic concentration of the ISF.

The contribution of urea to the countercurrent mechanism, whatever way it occurs, depends on the primary generating force for the mechanism, i.e., active transport of salt out of the thick ascending limb. This transport without water dilutes the tubular fluid flowing into the distal tubule and collecting tubule. The subsequent reabsorption of water in the cortex in response to this gradient raises the urea concentration in tubular fluid and begins to create the urea concentration gradient that drives urea reabsorption in the inner medullary segment of the collecting duct.

MEASUREMENT OF THE CONCENTRATING AND DILUTING ABILITY OF THE KIDNEY

The ability of the kidney to respond to dilution or concentration of the body's extracellular fluid (ECF) can be assessed qualitatively by measuring the urine osmotic concentration or the ratio of urine to plasma concentration, U_{Osm}/P_{Osm}. Normal humans can maximally concentrate their urine to 1200 to 1400 mOsm/kg H_2O. It is more accurate, however, to calculate the volume of water, free of solute, that is reabsorbed from the tubular fluid when the kidney is concentrating the urine or the volume of water free of solute that is retained within the urine when the kidney is diluting it. It is that volume of water that effectively changes the osmotic concentration of the ECF. The terms and simple equations that have been developed to calculate that volume are derived from an expression for solute or osmole clearance and a comparison of this to the urine flow rate. The clearance of solute particles from the plasma,

$$C_{Osm} = U_{Osm} \dot{V} / P_{Osm} \qquad \text{(ml/min)}$$

If the kidney reabsorbs water and solute in the same proportion as they exist in plasma, then the urine is isosmotic to plasma, $U_{Osm}/P_{Osm} = 1$, and solving the equation above, $C_{Osm} = \dot{V}$. In this situation, no change in the osmotic concentration of the ECF will result.

When ADH is present in the plasma in sufficient concentration, the kidney reabsorbs a greater percentage of the filtered water than of the filtered solute. A fraction of the water is reabsorbed free of the solute with which it was filtered, the urine is made hyperosmotic, $U_{Osm}/P_{Osm} > 1$ and $C_{Osm} > \dot{V}$. The difference between the actual urine flow and what it would have been if the urine were isosmotic is the volume of solute-free water reabsorbed, $T^c_{H_2O}$.

$$T^c_{H_2O} = C_{Osm} - \dot{V} \qquad \text{(ml/min)}$$

Consider for a moment that the kidney is excreting 1 ml/min of urine with an osmotic concentration of 580 μOsm/ml when the plasma osmotic concentration has risen slightly to 290 μOsm/ml.

$$T^c_{H_2O} = \frac{580 \ \mu\text{Osm/ml} \times 1 \ \text{ml/min}}{290 \ \mu\text{Osm/ml}} - 1 \ \text{ml/min} = 1 \ \text{ml/min}$$

The kidney is in effect reabsorbing the water from 1 ml/min of the filtrate and excreting the solute that was in it. That 1 ml/min of reabsorbed solute-free water is returned to the ECF which it dilutes. The reabsorption of solute-free water takes place in the medullary sections of the collecting ducts where the tubular fluid comes into contact with the hyperosmotic medullary ISF.

If ADH is absent and the kidney reabsorbs a smaller percentage of filtered water than solute, a fraction of the filtered water is excreted free of its solute. The urine is made hypo-osmotic: $U_{Osm}/P_{Osm} < 1$ and $C_{Osm} < \dot{V}$; the kidney is excreting more water than it would if the urine were isosmotic; and the difference is called the clearance of solute-free water, C_{H_2O}.

$$C_{H_2O} = \dot{V} - C_{Osm} \qquad \text{(ml/min)}$$

Consider now that the kidney is excreting 10 ml/min of urine with an osmotic concentration of 140 μOsm/ml. The plasma osmotic concentration is somewhat lower than normal, 280 μOsm/ml.

$$C_{H_2O} = 10 \ \text{ml/min} - \frac{140 \ \mu\text{Osm/ml} \times 10 \ \text{ml/min}}{280 \ \mu\text{Osm/ml}} = 5 \ \text{ml/min}$$

The kidney is now reabsorbing the solute from 5 ml/min of the filtrate and excreting the water. Solute-free water is removed from the ECF, thereby concentrating it.

FACTORS AFFECTING THE CONCENTRATING ABILITY OF THE KIDNEY

Anatomic

The longer the loops of Henle in proportion to the rest of the nephron, the greater the vertical interstitial osmotic gradient. Some mammals that live in a dry environment, such as the gerbil, the kangaroo rat, and the golden hamster, possess nephrons with loops so long that the papilla of these animals protrudes into the ureter. These animals may excrete urine with a concentration of 4000 to 5000 mOsm/kg H_2O. In contrast, the nephrons of beavers have short loops and their kidneys can only minimally concentrate the urine above the plasma level.

Physiologic

The antidiuretic hormone controls the permeability of the collecting tubules to water. If the hormone is present in reduced amounts or is absent, the permeability is decreased, the tubular fluid in the cortical sections of the collecting tubules does not come into osmotic equilibrium with the cortical interstitial fluid, and a large volume of hypoosmotic tubular fluid flows on into the medullary sections of the collecting tubules. Here also, the tubules' permeability to water is reduced and the urine does not become osmotically equilibrated with the medullary interstitial fluid. The osmotic concentration of the urine drops as solute reabsorption continues and water loss is increased.

Changes in the rate of blood flow through the vasa recta affect the rate at which it carries solute out of the medulla, and thereby affect the osmotic countercurrent gradient. It is difficult to assess the importance of this factor because no exact means of measuring this flow rate directly have been developed.

The flow rates through the loop of Henle and the collecting tubules and the ratio of these two flow rates affect the concentrating ability. To understand the effect of an increase in flow through the loop of Henle, one important facet of gradient-limited transport systems must be grasped. Figure 7-11A illustrates a small section of a hypothetical tubule immersed in a bath of infinite volume with a Na concentration of 150 mM. The tubule is relatively impermeable to water and possesses an active transport system for Na. As fluid flows through the tubule, the active transport system reduces the Na concentration in the tubular fluid. As that concentration falls, the rate of passive back-flux of Na into the tubule increases, and in this hypothetical tubule, the passive backflux rises to equal the rate of active transport out when the concentration falls to 60 mM. At that point no further net reabsorption of Na can occur. In Figure 7-11A, 90 μmoles of Na will be reabsorbed per minute before that point is reached. If the flow rate through the tubule is increased as in Figure 7-11B, the *amount* of Na flowing through the tubule per min doubles and the same rate of active transport out does not reduce the *concentration* of Na to the same extent. This keeps the rate of passive influx below the rate of the active outflux, and thus, the *net* rate of reabsorption increases. In reality, other factors limit the rate of increase in reabsorption, but the fact remains that a major limitation on these transport systems, the concentration gradient, permits a greater rate of reabsorption when the flow rate past them is increased.

An increase in flow rate through the loop of Henle occurs when GFR is increased or when reabsorption by the proximal tubule is reduced. The solute transport system in the ascending limb is thought to be gradient-limited. When the flow rate through this structure is raised, an increased amount of solute can be reabsorbed before the limiting gradient is reached. The deposition of this increased amount of solute into

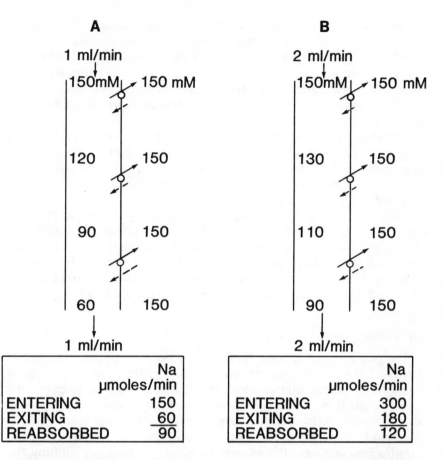

Figure 7-11. An illustration of the result of an increase in flow through a hypo-thetical tubular structure, poorly permeable to water and possessing a gradient-limited Na transport mechanism. As Na is actively transported out and the tubular fluid concen-tration drops, the rate of passive back-flux increases. In this hypothetical example, the rate of passive back-flux rises to equal the active transport rate when the tubular fluid concentration falls to 60 mM (as in A). At that point, no further net reabsorption can occur. If the flow rate through the tubule is doubled (as in B), the amount of Na entering the tubule per minute doubles and the same rate of active transport does not reduce the concentration of Na to the same extent. The passive back-flux rate is kept low, and thus the net rate of Na transport increases.

the finite volume of the medullary ISF augments the rate of water reab-sorption from the collecting tubules, that is, $T_{H_2O}^c$ rises.

If the volume flow into the medullary section of the collecting tubules rises, more water can be reabsorbed before the urine osmotic concentra-tion rises to the same level as that in the medullary ISF. For instance, if the flow rate into this section of the collecting tubules is 2 ml/min, the reabsorption of 1 ml/min of water will double its osmotic concentration.

If the flow rate into the tubules is increased to 4 ml/min, 2 ml/min can be reabsorbed before the osmotic concentration is doubled. However, this excess water entering the medullary ISF will dilute it and reduce the concentrating ability unless solute reabsorption from the ascending limb of Henle's loop is also increased. The flow rate into the collecting tubules may be raised by inhibition of solute reabsorption in the distal tubule and at other points upstream.

Maximum urine osmotic concentrations are achieved when the ratio of loop flow rate to collecting tubule flow rate is high. However, $T^c_{H_2O}$ is probably low when flow rate into the collecting tubule is low. $T^c_{H_2O}$ is high when a high loop flow occurs in conjunction with a moderate increase in collecting duct flow.

As has been explained, urea plays an important role in the countercurrent mechanism. Factors that influence the amount of urea in the glomerular filtrate affect the final osmotic concentration of the urine. One such factor is the amount of protein in the diet. An insufficient intake of protein reduces the effectiveness of the countercurrent mechanism and, thereby, the ability of an animal to cope with a low intake of water.

Pharmacologic

The primary driving force for the countercurrent system is the active transport of salt without water out of the ascending limb of the loop of Henle. Any agent that inhibits this transport system disrupts the countercurrent mechanism. Ethacrynic acid, furosemide, and to a lesser extent, the mercurial diuretics have this effect. Inhibition of solute reabsorption in the distal tubule increases the flow rate into the collecting tubules and increases the amount of water entering and diluting the medullary ISF. Amiloride, triamterene, and the thiazide diuretics may have this effect, so may aldosterone inhibitors. Other agents that primarily inhibit reabsorption in the proximal tubule increase volume flow into the loop of Henle and may increase $T^c_{H_2O}$.

It is important to realize that most diuretic agents probably affect reabsorption in all parts of the nephron to varying extents and their effect at any one site will be influenced by a variety of physiologic factors. Because of this, an analysis of their effect on the countercurrent system can be exceedingly complex. Drugs could inhibit the countercurrent system in other theoretical ways. Medullary blood flow could be altered and the effect of ADH could be modified.

Summary

The primary driving force causing the urine to become osmotically concentrated is the active transport of salt out of the ascending limb of the loop of Henle without concomitant water reabsorption. The resulting osmotic gradient established across the limb epithelium is "multiplied" and preserved by the countercurrent flows of urine in the loop of Henle and blood in the vasa recta, which serve to trap solute in the medulla and keep water out. In this way, a large vertical osmotic gradient is established down the length of the medulla, which then causes water to be reabsorbed from the collecting tubules. This last step only occurs in the presence of ADH, which controls the permeability of the collecting tubular epithelium to water.

BIBLIOGRAPHY

General:

See the following chapters from: Andreoli, T. E., Hoffman, J. F., and Fanestil, D. D., (Eds.): Physiology of Membrane Disorders. New York, Plenum Medical Book Co., 1978.
  Chapter 32. Giebisch, G.: The Proximal Nephron.
  Chapter 33. Burg, M. B., and Stephenson, J. L.: Transport Characteristics of the Loop of Henle.
  Chapter 34. Windhager, E. E., and Costanzo, L. S.: Transport Functions of the Distal Convoluted Tubule.
  Chapter 35. Schafer, J. A., and Andreoli, T. E.: The Collecting Duct.
See the following chapters from: Brenner, B. M. and Rector, F. C. Jr., (Eds.): The Kidney. 2nd ed. Philadelphia, W. B. Saunders Co., 1981.
  Chapter 7. Burg, M. B.: Renal Handling of Sodium Chloride, Water, Amino Acids and Glucose.
  Chapter 11. Jamison, R. L.: Urine Concentration and Dilution.

Specific:

Andreoli, T. E., and Schafer, J. A.: Effective lumenal hypotonicity: the driving force for isotonic proximal tubular fluid absorption. Am. J. Physiol., 236 (Renal Fluid Electrolyte Physiol. 5): F89, 1979.
Andreoli, T. E., Berliner, R. W., Kokko, J. P., and Marsh, D. J.: Questions and replies: renal mechanisms for urinary concentrating and diluting ability. Am. J. Physiol. 235 (Renal Fluid Electrolyte Physiol. 4): F1, 1978.
Frizzell, R. A., Field, M., and Schultz, S. G.: Sodium-coupled chloride transport by epithelial tissues. Am. J. Physiol., 236 (Renal Fluid Electrolyte Physiol. 5): F1, 1979.
Jorgensen, P. L.: Sodium and potassium ion pump in kidney tubules. Physiol. Rev., 60:864, 1980.
Schafer, J. A., and Andreoli, T. E.: Rheogenic and passive Na^+ absorption by the proximal nephron. Ann. Rev. Physiol., 41:211, 1979.
Ullrich, K. J.: Sugar, amino acid, and Na^+ cotransport in the proximal tubule. Ann. Rev. Physiol., 41:181, 1979.

CHAPTER 8

Diuresis

The preceding chapter described the tubular reabsorptive mechanisms that conserve salt and water. This chapter describes how inhibition of the reabsorptive mechanisms causes diuresis, that is, increased excretion of water and solute.

There are two types of diuresis. One is water diuresis, in which there is an increase in water excretion but little or no increase in solute excretion. The primary cause is an excessive intake of water or inhibition of water reabsorption in collecting tubules. The second type is solute or osmotic diuresis in which both solute and water excretion increase. This can be caused by an increased intake of solute or by inhibition of solute reabsorption, both of which lead to an indirect inhibition of water reabsorption.

WATER DIURESIS

Water diuresis usually results from a fall in the plasma concentration of ADH. The lack of ADH causes the collecting tubular epithelium to lose its permeability to water and water reabsorption is reduced despite the presence of high osmotic pressure gradients across the epithelium. However, solute reabsorption continues, so solute is removed from the water in the tubular fluid and solute-free water is excreted, or in other words, solute-free water is cleared (C_{H_2O}) from the extracellular fluid.

ADH does not affect proximal tubular reabsorption. Thus, water diuresis is the result of inhibition of water reabsorption in only the distal sections of the nephron. The maximum urine volume in water diuresis never exceeds 8 to 11% of the GFR. However, this is equivalent to a urine flow approaching 20 L or 5 gal per day when the diuresis is sustained.

SOLUTE DIURESIS

Solute diuresis can be caused by the presence in the glomerular filtrate of solutes in large excess of the amount the tubule can reabsorb or by the inhibition of specific reabsorptive mechanisms. In either situation, the reabsorption of many other solutes is reduced and water reabsorption falls. Urine volume rises and the osmotic concentration of the urine declines toward the plasma level. In most situations, reabsorption of fluid in the proximal tubule is affected and the increased flow of tubular fluid into the rest of the nephron affects reabsorption there. Often, distal sections of the nephron are also primarily affected. More rarely, reabsorption in the distal sections only may be inhibited.

In order to explain solute diuresis, the limitations and interdependence of the reabsorptive processes in the proximal tubule must first be restated. Since the proximal tubular epithelium is highly permeable to water, the tubular fluid always remains isosmotic with the interstitial fluid surrounding the tubule. Therefore, water can be reabsorbed only when solute is reabsorbed and the two must be reabsorbed in the same proportion as they exist in the tubular fluid; that is, the reabsorbed fluid must also be isosmotic. Thus, reabsorption of water in the proximal tubule is limited by the extent to which all the various solutes are reabsorbed. Any reduction in solute reabsorption in the proximal tubule produces an equivalent effect on water reabsorption. The chief osmotic solutes in the filtrate are Na and its attendant anions. These are extensively reabsorbed by gradient-limited transport systems. The tubular epithelium is so permeable to Na, however, that if water reabsorption is retarded for some reason and active reabsorption of Na begins to reduce the Na concentration, the passive back-flux of Na into the tubule quickly rises and the net reabsorptive flux falls to zero. In other words, the proximal tubule can reabsorb salt only to the extent that it reabsorbs water. Because of this close interrelationship between salt and water transport, the reabsorption of both can be blocked by inhibiting the reabsorption of either.

Let us consider first how water reabsorption can be primarily inhibited and how this secondarily inhibits salt reabsorption. Normally, a small fraction of the solute present in the glomerular filtrate is poorly reabsorbed by the proximal tubule. As the reabsorption of the other solutes and water proceeds, the concentration of these nonreabsorbable solutes in the tubular fluid increases. Since the total solute concentration must always remain the same, reabsorption will continue only to the extent that the concentration of other solutes can be reduced. The proximal tubule can do this to some extent. For example, the concentration of glucose in the tubular fluid is reduced essentially to zero. However, the concentration of the major osmotic solutes in the tubular fluid, Na and its attendant anions, can be reduced only slightly. Therefore, as the reabsorption of fluid raises the concentration of nonreabsorbable solute in the filtrate, a point is reached at which the Na concentration must be reduced if the total osmotic concentration of the tubular fluid is to be maintained constant and water reabsorption is to proceed. Since the Na concentration can be reduced only to a small extent, water and salt reabsorption are halted soon after that point is reached.

Table 8-1 illustrates how this principle works in the normal situation and the consequences of an increase in the plasma concentration of nonreabsorbable solute. In the normal situation, the concentration of nonreabsorbable solute in plasma and thus in the glomerular filtrate is low. Its concentration in tubular fluid is doubled when 50% of the filtrate is reabsorbed, but this can be balanced by a fall in the concentration of glucose, amino acids, and other substances as they are reabsorbed. In this way, the total osmotic concentration of the filtrate stays constant. Additional fluid can be reabsorbed beyond that point as the concentration of glucose, amino acids, and others are reduced further. When the concentration of nonreabsorbable solute in the plasma is increased, however, 50% of the filtrate can be reabsorbed in the example shown only if the concentrations of glucose, amino acids, and others fall towards zero and the concentration of Na is reduced also.

TABLE 8-1   AN ILLUSTRATION OF THE EFFECT OF NONREABSORB-ABLE SOLUTE ON PROXIMAL TUBULAR REABSORPTION OF WATER AND SALT.

Nonreabsorbable Solute	Solute Concentrations, mOsm/kg H_2O Glucose, amino acids, etc.	Inorganic ions	Total
I. Normal Situation			
a. In the glomerular filtrate:			
3	7	280	290
b. In the proximal tubular fluid after reabsorption of 50% of the filtrate:			
6	4	280	290
c. After reabsorption of 70%:			
10	0	280	290
II. After accumulation of nonreabsorbable solute in the plasma			
a. In the glomerular filtrate:			
15	7	280	302
b. In the proximal tubular fluid after reabsorption of 50% of the filtrate:			
30	0	272	302

(The concentrations listed here are approximations only.)

The depression in proximal tubular reabsorption increases the volume flow into the distal sections of the nephron. The effect of changes in flow rate through the medullary sections of the nephron was described in detail in the previous chapter. When the flow rate rises, the amount of salt flowing into these sections of the nephrons increases, but the salt concentration of the fluid does not change. This permits the gradient-limited transport mechanisms to reabsorb a greater amount of salt before the gradient-limiting concentrations are reached (see Fig. 7-11). Thus, the inhibition of salt reabsorption in the proximal tubule is partly counteracted by increased reabsorption in the more distal segments of the nephron. This is not complete however, and the amount of salt excreted also rises.

When the volume of water flowing into the collecting tubule increases, the amount of water that is reabsorbed there rises. There are two reasons for this. Water moves out of the collecting tubule in response to the higher osmotic concentration in the interstitial fluid surrounding the tubule both in the cortex and in the medulla. Water reabsorption ceases only when the osmotic concentration of the tubular fluid rises to equal that of the interstitial fluid. Thus, an increase in the volume of hypotonic fluid flowing through the tubule permits a rise in the amount of water that can be reabsorbed before osmotic equilibration between the tubular fluid and the interstitial fluid occurs. In addition, the increased amount of solute transported into the medulla by the loop of Henle also enables additional water to be reabsorbed from the collecting tubule. As with salt, the inhibition of water reabsorption in the proximal tubule is partly, but not completely, counteracted by this increased reabsorption in the more distal segments of the nephron, and the rate of water excretion also rises. It is possible in extreme situations to depress proximal reabsorption to such an extent that the volume flow through the rest of the nephron becomes great. In this situation, the amount of salt and water reabsorbed in the distal sections of the nephron is disproportionately small in relation to the flow rate, the countercurrent system is overwhelmed, the medullary osmotic gradient is lost, and solute-free water reabsorption is reduced. The composition of the urine then begins to resemble that of the glomerular filtrate.

Urea is one solute that can cause primary inhibition of water reabsorption. Urea is reabsorbed to some extent by the proximal tubule, but its concentration does rise in the tubular fluid as water is reabsorbed. This rise in concentration must be balanced by a fall in the concentration of some other solute if the total solute concentration is to remain constant and water reabsorption is to continue. A rise in the plasma concentration of urea, such as may occur in a person on a high protein diet, will cause a mild solute diuresis. Mannitol, a monosaccharide resembling glucose, is often used to produce solute or osmotic diuresis. Mannitol is not metabolized by the body and is poorly reabsorbed by the nephron.

It is much more effective than urea in causing diuresis because the tubule is much less permeable to it. Glucose also causes solute diuresis when it is present in the glomerular filtrate in a quantity that exceeds the Tm of the glucose transport system. This may occur in uncontrolled diabetes mellitus.

Primary inhibition of solute transport systems by pharmacologic agents causes a secondary inhibition of water reabsorption and the same general type of diuresis described earlier will ensue. For instance, acetazolamide inhibits bicarbonate reabsorption, particularly in the proximal tubule. The drop in anion reabsorption retards Na reabsorption and this secondarily blocks water reabsorption. Many of the diuretic agents used clinically inhibit active transport of salt primarily, and by doing so, inhibit water reabsorption. The characteristics of drug-induced diuresis may differ somewhat from the diuresis produced by urea or by mannitol. The more commonly used drugs have a major effect on salt reabsorption in the loop of Henle or on more distal segments of the nephron. Any inhibition of proximal reabsorption that may occur is probably a minor factor in the total diuresis (see Chapter 13).

Alterations in the physiologic factors controlling salt and water reabsorption also cause solute diuresis. For instance, a fall in the colloid osmotic pressure of plasma in the peritubular capillary will reduce reabsorption in the proximal tubule and increase the flow rate into the rest of the nephron. A rise in GFR will also increase volume flow into the distal sections of the nephron. In some of these situations, reabsorption by these segments may increase and blunt the diuresis to some extent, as has been described. In other situations, reabsorption in the distal structures is also inhibited.

BIBLIOGRAPHY

Burg, M. B.: Renal Handling of Sodium Chloride, Water, Amino Acids and Glucose. *In* The Kidney. 2nd ed. Edited by B. M. Brenner, and F. C. Rector Jr., Philadelphia W. B. Saunders Co., 1981.

Grantham, J. J., and Chonko, A. M.: The Physiological Basis and Clinical Use of Diuretics. *In* Sodium and Water Homeostasis. Edited by B. M. Brenner, and J. H. Stein, Contempory Issues in Nephrology. Vol. 1. New York, Churchill Livingstone, 1978.

CHAPTER *9*

Control of Osmotic Concentration and Volume of Extracellular Fluid

REGULATION OF THE OSMOTIC CONCENTRATION

The osmotic pressure of the extracellular fluid is maintained at a constant level primarily by regulation of water excretion through the action of antidiuretic hormone (ADH). ADH, also called vasopressin, is an octapeptide that is produced in the magnocellular system of the hypothalamus, specifically within cells of the supraoptic and paraventricular nuclei. The hormone is synthesized and packaged in neurosecretory granules with a protein, neurophysin. The granules flow along the axons of these cells to the nerve endings in the posterior pituitary where they are stored. ADH is released from the nerve endings by exocytosis in response to stimulation of the neurons.

Control of ADH Secretion

A negative-feedback reflex mechanism regulates the osmotic concentration of the ECF by controlling the secretion of ADH (Fig. 9-1). The stimulus is a rise in ECF osmotic concentration. The sensors are osmoreceptors located in the anterior hypothalamus near the neurons that manufacture ADH. These receptors are thought to be sensitive to changes in their intracellular volume or osmotic concentration caused by changes in the effective osmotic concentration of the fluid surrounding them. Axons of the receptors evidently impinge on the secretory neurons, and impulses are transmitted from the receptors to the secretory neuron endings in the posterior pituitary. The released ADH triggers increased water reabsorption. This, coupled with continued solute excretion, reduces the osmotic concentration of the ECF, providing the negative feedback to the osmoreceptors that induces a fall in the rate of ADH release.

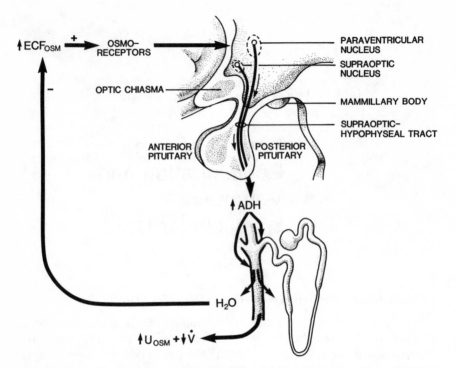

Figure 9-1. The negative feedback mechanism that regulates the osmotic concentration of the extracellular fluid (ECF_{osm}).

The relationship between the plasma or ECF osmotic concentrations and the plasma concentration of ADH is illustrated in Figure 9-2. At osmotic concentrations below 280 mOsm/kg H_2O, the level of ADH in plasma is relatively constant at about 0.5 picograms/ml (pg/ml, 10^{-12} g/ml). When plasma osmolality rises above that threshold concentration of about 280 mOsm/kg H_2O, ADH secretion is stimulated. The maximally effective concentration of ADH, that is, the concentration that brings about the maximum urine osmotic concentration, is reached when the plasma osmotic concentration rises to 294 to 295 mOsm/kg H_2O.

Figure 9-3 illustrates the relationship between the stimulus (plasma osmotic concentration), the effector (plasma ADH concentration), and the response, (changes in urine osmotic concentration and urine flow). The range of plasma osmotic concentration that can change plasma ADH concentration from the threshold level to the maximum effective concentration is only 15 mOsm/kg H_2O, from 280 to 295 mOsm/kg H_2O. This small variation in plasma osmolality acting through the ADH mechanism can cause the urine osmotic concentration and flow rate to vary from 50 mOsm/kg H_2O and 20 L/day to 1200 mOsm/kg H_2O and 0.8

L/day. (It should be realized that changes in the rate of solute excretion can alter the urine flow rate and osmotic concentration normally present at any given level of plasma ADH concentration.) The exquisite sensitivity of this feedback mechanism is such that a change in 1% in the plasma osmotic concentration (~3 mOsm/kg H_2O) causes a change in plasma ADH concentration of 1 pg/ml, which is sufficient to alter urine osmolality by about 250 mOsm/kg H_2O. In an individual weighing 70 kg, this change can be produced by drinking 400 to 450 ml or 14 oz of water.

In normal individuals, the basal plasma osmotic concentration averages about 287 mOsm/kg H_2O. This maintains a plasma ADH concentration between 2 and 2.5 pg/ml, which in turn, results in a urine osmotic

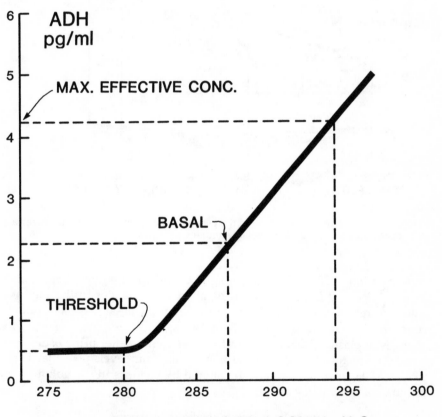

Figure 9-2. The relation between the plasma osmotic concentration and the plasma ADH concentration. The maximum effective concentration is that which causes the kidney to maximally concentrate the urine. (Adapted from a figure in: Robertson, G. L., Mahr, E. A., Athar, S., and Sinha, T.: Development and clinical application of a new method for the radioimmunoassay of arginine vasopressin in human plasma. J. Clin. Invest., 52:2340, 1973.)

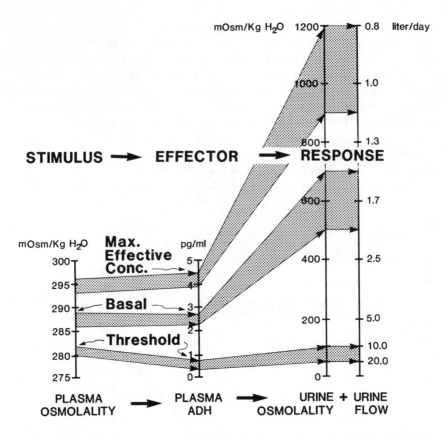

Figure 9-3. The relationship among the plasma osmotic concentration, the plasma ADH concentration, and urine osmolality and flow rate.

concentration of 500 to 700 mOsm/kg H_2O and a urine flow of approximately 1.4 to 2.0 L/day. This can be altered by changes in the rate of solute excretion caused by other factors. From the basal plasma osmotic concentration a rise or fall of 7 mOsm/kg H_2O (~2.5%) results in changes in plasma ADH concentration sufficient to alter urine osmolality and urine flow to the minimum and maximum levels possible. The rate of ADH secretion can also be altered by changes in the volume of plasma, as will be discussed.

Sequence of Events in Response to Intake of Water.

Consider a subject weighing 70 kg who ingests 1 L of water containing no solute. As the water is absorbed into the blood from the gastrointestinal tract, it passes by osmosis into both the extracellular and intracellular water compartments, reducing the osmotic concentration of both compartments to the same level. Cells contain 72% of total body water. Thus, cells also contain 72% of the osmotically active solute. Therefore, in diluting both compartments to the same concentration, 720 ml of the ingested water will enter the intracellular compartment and 280 ml will remain in the extracellular space. This is a small increase in the volume of the ECF (2.5%) and only a small fraction of that remains in plasma. It is probably not large enough to trigger any of the reflex mechanisms controlling the volume of the ECF; nor is it large enough to alter the blood pressure or the colloid osmotic pressure of the plasma. Thus, there is no change in GFR.

There is, however, a small but distinct drop in the osmotic concentration of the body water of about 7 mOsm/kg H_2O or 2.5%. Theoretically, the osmoreceptors in the hypothalamus should expand as they take in water, causing them to inhibit ADH release from the posterior pituitary. Within 15 to 20 minutes, this drop in secretion, together with the continued metabolism and excretion of circulating ADH, causes a drop in its plasma concentration. The collecting tubules then begin to lose their permeability to water and the urine flow begins to rise and reaches a peak of approximately 15 ml/min in 60 to 90 minutes. As water is excreted, the osmotic concentration of the ECF begins to rise, water begins to leave the body cells, including osmoreceptors, and ADH secretion begins to rise. In 120 to 150 minutes, the urine flow returns to the control level. By that time, almost all the ingested fluid has been excreted. During this period, there has been no change in GFR and little change in solute excretion. The major change has been in water excretion and the major reason for that change has been the fall in the plasma concentration of ADH.

Mechanism of Action of ADH

ADH specifically binds to receptors in the basolateral membranes of cells in the latter portion of the distal tubules and in the collecting tubules (Fig. 9-4). This coupling of receptor and ADH activates adenyl cyclase, which catalyzes the production of cyclic adenosine monophosphate (cyclic AMP). It is the increased concentration of this "second messenger" within the cell that ultimately leads to increased water flow through the apical membrane of the cell. Cyclic AMP is broken down to 5' AMP by phosphodiesterase (PDIE).

The mechanism by which increased cell concentrations of cyclic AMP stimulate water flow is not completely delineated. It is probable that cyclic AMP activates a protein kinase enzyme which catalyzes the transfer of phosphorus from ATP onto side chains of polypeptides. The nature of these polypeptides is not known for certain. However, it has recently become apparent that ADH-induced water flow depends on the integrity of cytoplasmic microtubules (MT) and microfilaments (MF). Microtubules are linear, unbranched structures with a diameter of about 250 Å that are polymerized from a soluble protein called tubulin. Micro-

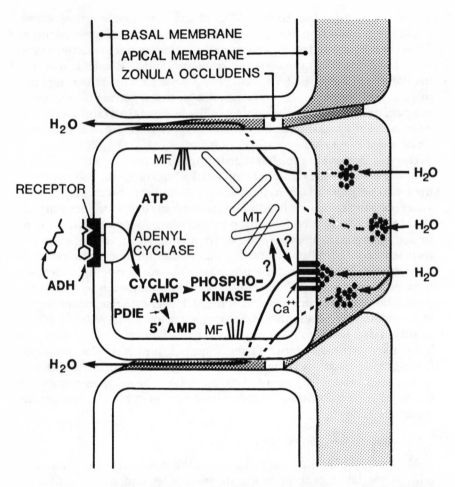

Figure 9-4. The effect of ADH on distal tubule and collecting duct cells. Parts of the depicted mechanism are hypothetical. PDIE = phosphodiesterase, MF = microfilaments, MT = microtubules. (Adapted from figures in: Dousa, T. P., and Valtin, H.: Cellular actions of vasopressin in the mammalian kidney. Kidney Internat. *10:*46, 1976; and Hays, R. M., and Levine, S. D.: Pathophysiology of water metabolism. *In* Brenner, B. M., and Rector, F. C., Jr. (eds): The Kidney. 2nd Ed. Philadelphia, W. B. Saunders Co., 1981.)

filaments are fibrous linear structures with a diameter of about 50 Å. They are composed of proteins with biochemical properties similar to those of muscle actin.

The relationships among protein kinase, microtubules, microfilaments, and changes in water flow across the apical membrane are not understood; it has been observed however, that, following the application of ADH to the basal surface of sensitive cells, tightly packed aggregates of intramembranous particles appear in the apical membrane. It is thought that calcium is required for these aggregates to form. The structure of these aggregates and their relationship to microtubules or microfilaments or even to cyclic AMP are not known. It is believed that these "patches" or aggregates on the apical membrane surface provide an area of high water permeability for the diffusion of water. Although this action of ADH permits a high rate of water diffusion, the net movement of water out of the lumen also requires the establishment of an osmotic pressure gradient. This is the function of the countercurrent system and the solute transport mechanisms.

Several disorders of the ADH system have been recognized. The syndrome of diabetes insipidus is characterized by the excretion of large quantities of dilute urine. This may be due to a primary insufficiency of ADH, related to dysfunction or loss of function of the hypothalamic-neurohypophyseal tract; an inability of the kidney to respond to ADH (nephrogenic diabetes insipidus); or a psychogenic disorder causing compulsive water drinking (polydipsia), which physiologically reduces the secretion of ADH. The first type can be successfully treated with synthetic analogs of antidiuretic hormone, which have greater antidiuretic potency and much less vasopressor activity than ADH. One of these is desmopressin (1-desamino-8-D-arginine vasopressin).

Excessive secretion of ADH may occur in patients with a variety of tumors, head injuries, or other diseases. This is called the syndrome of inappropriate secretion of ADH (SIADH). The excessive effect of ADH can be antagonized by lithium carbonate or by the antibiotic demeclocycline.

CONTROL OF EXTRACELLULAR FLUID VOLUME

The extracellular fluid compartment is a complex entity composed not only of two major divisions, the vascular and the interstitial fluid compartments, but also of several subdivisions of these, each with differing characteristics. It is not surprising, therefore, that the control of ECF fluid volume, in marked contrast to control of the ECF osmotic concentration, is accomplished by a variety of mechanisms, many of which are poorly understood.

It is customary to speak of control of extracellular fluid volume, but it is apparent that the various mechanisms are triggered by factors related to the volume of the vascular compartment. Changes in the volume of the interstitial compartment ordinarily take place indirectly as a result of changes in the dynamic steady state of the Starling forces governing fluid movement across capillary walls separating the vascular and interstitial compartments.

The osmotic control mechanism and the various volume control mechanisms would often conflict with one another if both operated to control water excretion directly. Instead, the volume control mechanisms operate primarily by controlling the amount of the principal osmotic constituent present in the extracellular fluid, NaCl. Alterations induced in the excretion of NaCl by these mechanisms tend to cause the retention or excretion of an osmotic equivalent of water either directly, through the influence of salt reabsorption on water reabsorption, or indirectly, through the influence of changes in the NaCl concentration of the ECF on osmotic concentration and the secretion of ADH.

VASCULAR COMPARTMENTS AND VOLUME RECEPTORS

The volume of the vascular compartment can be divided into two sections, the high pressure arterial compartment and the low pressure venous compartment which includes the pulmonary circulation and all the heart except for the left ventricle (Fig. 9-5). The volume of the arterial compartment is primarily a direct function of the inflow, that is, the cardiac output, and the outflow, which is governed by arterial pressure and peripheral resistance. The compliance or distensibility of the muscular arterial wall is normally a minor factor. Changes in the volume of the arterial compartment are sensed primarily as changes in pressure by baroreceptors in the carotid sinus and aortic arch and by an intrarenal baroreceptor.

The volume of the venous compartment is primarily a direct function of the inflow, which is controlled by arterial pressure and total peripheral resistance, the outflow, and to a major extent, the venous compliance. The major factor controlling compliance is the tissue pressure exerted on the wall of the veins. It is also partially controlled by the activity of venous smooth muscle. In muscles of the trunk and the extremities, the tissue pressure is the result of the muscular contraction which compresses the veins and reduces their capacity. In the abdomen, contraction of the diaphragm and abdominal muscles compresses the abdominal veins. Most importantly, in the thorax, contraction of the rib muscles and diaphragm expands the thorax and reduces intrathoracic pressure, increasing the capacity of the great veins, the pulmonary circulation, and the atria. The atria and great veins in particular are highly distensible: small increases in transmural pressure produce large changes in their volume. Changes in volume stimulate stretch receptors (baroreceptors) embedded in the wall of these vessels. These receptors are known to exist in the wall of the left atrium and may exist also in the walls of the great veins and in the pulmonary circulation. In addition, volume receptors may exist in the hepatic circulation.

The volume of the interstitial compartment changes primarily as a result of changes in the balance between the capillary hydrostatic pressure (P_c) and the colloid osmotic pressure of the blood (π_b) (Fig. 9-5). A fall in peripheral resistance increases the pressure transmitted into the capillaries and causes a shift of isotonic fluid into the interstitial com-

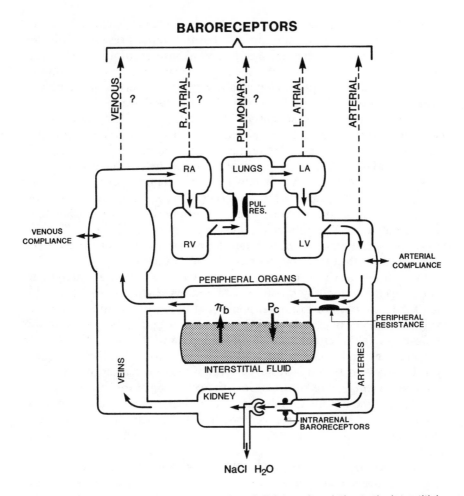

Figure 9-5. The vascular compartment, its subdivisions, its relation to the interstitial compartment, and the location of baroreceptors. RA and LA = right and left atria. RV and LV = right and left ventricles. π_b = colloid osmotic pressure of blood, P_c = capillary hydrostatic pressure.

partment. An increase in venous volume and pressure may be transmitted backward into the capillaries and have the same effect. An excessive intake of salt and water will not only increase P_c but will also reduce π_b by dilution, causing a major fraction of the excessive intake to be deposited in the interstitial space. Other more unusual changes alter the dynamic relationship between the volumes of the vascular and interstitial compartments. The leakage of protein into the interstitial space decreases the effective π_b and can cause a net shift of fluid into the interstitial space. Starvation or the loss of plasma proteins, such as in the nephrotic syndrome, has the same effect.

A fall in the volume of the vascular compartment caused by NaCl depletion or by hemorrhage causes a fall in arterial pressure. This decreases the activity of arterial and intrarenal baroreceptors. Venous volume decreases and reduces the activity of stretch receptors. The fall in activity of these receptors activates a variety of effector mechanisms, which decrease salt and H_2O excretion by the kidney. In addition, peripheral resistance is increased. The resulting fall in P_c causes a net shift of fluid from the interstitial space into the vascular compartment.

Expansion of the vascular compartment primarily increases venous volume and stimulates stretch receptors in the distensible thoracic vessels and atria. Arterial baroreceptors are stimulated not so much by an increase in arterial volume but by a rise in arterial pressure caused by an increase in cardiac output. Again, a variety of effector mechanisms are activated, leading to increased excretion of salt and water. The rise in venous pressure and fall in arteriolar resistance raises P_c and causes a net shift of fluid into the interstitial compartment.

In addition to these changes in total vascular volume, changes in effective circulating blood volume can be caused without directly altering total volume. For example, pooling of blood in leg and abdominal veins as a result of gravity during quiet standing may be sensed in the thorax as a fall in circulating blood volume, and this activates efferent mechanisms that decrease salt and water excretion. Conflicting signals can be received by the arterial and venous baroreceptors in some instances. In congestive failure or in severe stenosis of the mitral or aortic valves, cardiac output is reduced and arterial pressure falls, reducing stimulation of arterial baroreceptors. The fall in cardiac output, however, causes venous and atrial volume to expand, stimulating stretch receptors.

The exact response of any one of the known and postulated baroreceptors to a particular change in vascular volume is poorly documented and the efferent path or paths activated by any one set of baroreceptors is not fully delineated, except perhaps, for the intrarenal baroreceptor. Therefore, it is difficult to describe discrete feedback mechanisms. One must simply describe the afferent baroreceptors more or less as a group, and separately list effector mechanisms that may be triggered by stimulation or inhibition of one or more of the baroreceptors.

ROLE OF THE JUXTAGLOMERULAR APPARATUS

The juxtaglomerular apparatus receives and processes a variety of signals arising from changes in vascular volume and effects changes in salt and water excretion (Fig. 9-6). It is a primary receiver of information: the afferent arteriole, acting as a baroreceptor, can directly alter renin release in response to changes in arterial pressure. This is the intrarenal baroreceptor that was referred to earlier. In addition, changes in the rate of delivery of fluid to the macula densa via the tubule can also

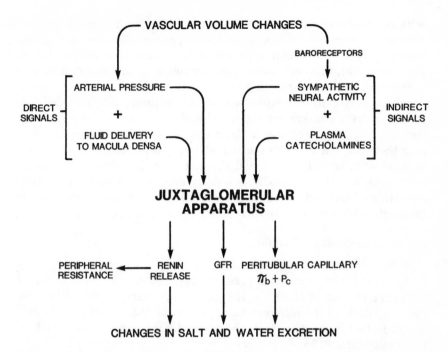

Figure 9-6. The signals that impinge upon the juxtaglomerular apparatus in response to vascular volume changes and the effector mechanisms controlled by the apparatus.

alter the rate of renin release. The juxtaglomerular apparatus is also a secondary receiver of information. Neural and humoral factors triggered by changes in stimulation of other baroreceptors impinge upon it.

The apparatus responds to these signals in a variety of ways to induce changes in salt and water excretion. The rate of release of renin can be altered, GFR can be changed, and the balance between hydrostatic pressure and colloid osmotic pressure in the peritubular capillaries can be shifted, thereby causing a change in salt and water excretion from the nephron. In addition, the release of renin can serve to alter vascular volume by increasing peripheral resistance.

EFFECTOR MECHANISMS

GFR

Normally, the filtration rate is autoregulated within a narrow range. In some instances, however, the autoregulatory mechanisms can be overridden by external signals received by the juxtaglomerular apparatus (Chapter 4). The fall in arterial pressure following hemorrhage, for example, reduces the inhibition of sympathetic nervous system activity by arterial baroreceptors. The resulting increase in renal neural activity and circulating catecholamines can cause arteriolar constriction within the juxtaglomerular apparatus which will reduce RBF and GFR. The fall in filtration rate reduces the excretion of salt and water, thus conserving extracellular fluid volume.

Following significant expansion of ECF volume, RBF and GFR are increased by an unknown mechanism, but the extent to which the increase in GFR contributes to the increase in salt and water excretion may be small. The rate of tubular reabsorption of salt and water tends to increase when GFR rises, and the increment in excretion is a small fraction of the increase in GFR. In volume expansion, other mechanisms are activated that reduce salt and water reabsorption (vide infra). These evidently are primarily responsible for the resulting diuresis.

Peritubular Capillary Pressures

In the peritubular capillaries, the colloid osmotic pressure (π_b) normally exceeds the hydrostatic pressure (P_c), facilitating reabsorption of fluid from the proximal tubule. The level of π_b is partially determined by the magnitude of the filtration fraction, that is, the fraction of protein-free fluid that is removed from the plasma at the glomerulus (filtration fraction = GFR/RPF). P_c is altered by changes in constriction in the afferent and efferent arterioles (Chapter 7). Following blood volume expansion, the rise in RBF may be greater than the increase in GFR (Fig. 9-7). Consequently, the filtration fraction, and thus π_b, falls. At the same time, the dilitation of the arterioles that produced the increase in RBF causes a rise in P_c downstream from the arterioles. These two changes cause the net force for fluid reabsorption from the paracellular spaces into the capillary to decrease (Fig. 7-5). This results in increased back-flux of salt and water from the paracellular space through the zonula occludens into the proximal tubular lumen. Conversely, in volume depletion, the fall in RPF may exceed the decrease in GFR. This results in an increase in π_b. At the same time, the constriction of the arterioles upstream causes P_c to fall. These changes combine to increase the net driving force for fluid movement from the paracellular space into the capillary.

Renin, Angiotensin, Aldosterone

The renin-angiotensin-aldosterone axis plays an important role in the control of ECF volume and blood pressure. Angiotensin serves as a primary effector in that it causes vasoconstriction. It also stimulates aldosterone synthesis by the adrenal cortex. Other possible effects of angiotensin include stimulation of thirst, ADH secretion, the sympathetic nervous system, and Na reabsorption. It has recently been discovered that all the components required for angiotensin genera-

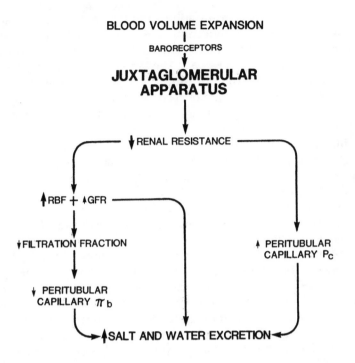

Figure 9-7. The effect of blood volume expansion on pressures in the peritubular capillaries.

tion exist in brain tissue. This intriguing finding has many possible implications.

Aldosterone is an important factor in the body's response to a fall in ECF volume. Its stimulation of sodium reabsorption has a direct effect at the tubular level of increasing water reabsorption, and by promoting the retention of salt, it may increase the osmotic concentration of the ECF, thereby stimulating ADH secretion and causing a further increase in water reabsorption.

The major factor controlling aldosterone secretion is the plasma concentration of angiotensin II, which in turn, is controlled by the rate of renin secretion. Angiotensin II stimulates the zona glomerulosa of the adrenal cortex to produce aldosterone. The heptapeptide angiotensin III is also a potent stimulus of aldosterone secretion. The subsequent increase in salt and water reabsorption tends to increase ECF volume, which, acting through the renin system, exerts a negative feedback influence on plasma angiotensin II concentration.

Other factors also influence aldosterone secretion. The plasma Na concentration may exert a controlling influence directly on the adrenal cortex; a decrease in Na concentration stimulates aldosterone secretion. High plasma potassium concentrations also directly stimulate the adrenal cortex to release aldosterone. Aldosterone has the additional effect of promoting K secretion. The adrenocorticotropic hormone (ACTH) secreted by the anterior pituitary also plays a role. It does not serve to control closely the rate of secretion but rather exerts a permissive effect: Its presence is necessary for aldosterone secretion to increase in response to other stimuli.

The juxtaglomerular apparatus is the major receptor controlling the rate of aldosterone secretion through its influence on the plasma concentration of angiotensin. Three major stimuli induce the juxtaglomerular apparatus to release renin (Fig. 9-8): a fall in arterial pressure, acting directly on the intrarenal baroreceptor, the afferent arteriole; an increase in sympathetic neural and humoral activity, acting through β_2 receptors; and a decrease in the rate of delivery of fluid to the macula densa cells by the tubule. The fall in fluid delivery can be caused by a decrease in GFR following the fall in arterial pressure and activation of the sympathetic nervous system. An increase in reabsorption by the proximal tubule can have the same effect. The exact nature of the signal to the macula densa and how it is transmitted to the granular cells is in doubt. The signal may be the amount of sodium or chloride that is delivered to the macula densa. Usually, this is a function of the tubular fluid flow rate.

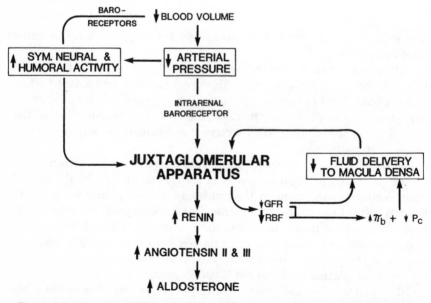

Figure 9-8. The three factors that act upon the juxtaglomerular apparatus to increase the secretion of aldosterone when blood volume is reduced.

The connection between the role of the macula densa in controlling renin secretion and its role in the autoregulation of GFR, described in Chapter 4, is not understood.

The mechanism of action of aldosterone is only partially understood. The hormone combines with a receptor in the cytoplasm of distal tubular and collecting duct cells. The steroid-receptor complex then interacts with chromatin in the nucleus to increase the formation of messenger RNA and ribosomal RNA. These increase the synthesis of specific proteins. The role of these proteins is not known for certain. At least three specific changes in the cell have been identified: The permeation of Na into the cell through the apical membrane is increased, the activity of Na-K-ATPase rises, and mitochondrial enzymes involved in oxidative metabolism are increased. Which, if any, of these effects is primary is not known.

The response to a rise in plasma aldosterone levels requires one to two hours to become apparent. Thus aldosterone plays only a limited role in the response of the kidney to acute changes in ECF fluid volume. It is an important factor, however, in the long term response to alterations in ECF volume. High aldosterone levels may also be the primary factor in most chronic states of salt retention.

A phenomemon called "mineralocorticoid escape" has been recognized and investigated recently. Simply, it is the type of response seen in an organism when one variable is subject to more than one control mechanism. A rise in plasma aldosterone level, usually due to a tumor in the zona glomerulosa of an adrenal gland, induces the retention of salt, i.e., the rate of salt excretion becomes less than the rate of intake (Fig. 9-9). This causes ECF volume to increase over a period of days, until other mechanisms that respond to changes in ECF volume are triggered (GFR, peritubular capillary pressures, and the like). Salt excretion then increases ("escapes"), despite continued high levels of aldosterone, until a balanced state is achieved. The ECF volume then stabilizes at a steady state level higher than that which existed prior to the rise in aldosterone. (The "braking" phenomenon described in Chapter 13 is the obverse of this type of response.) Patients with congestive heart failure or liver failure also may have high plasma levels of aldosterone, but in these conditions (secondary hyperaldosteronism), in contrast to adrenal cortical tumors (primary aldosteronism), salt is persistently retained. In other words, the organism fails to "escape" from the sodium retention caused by aldosterone.

Renal Nerves

The sympathetic neural innervation of the kidney can alter renin release, GFR, and RPF, as described earlier. In addition, it has been discovered that sympathetic adrenergic fibers reach the basement membrane of proximal and distal tubules and that stimulation of the renal

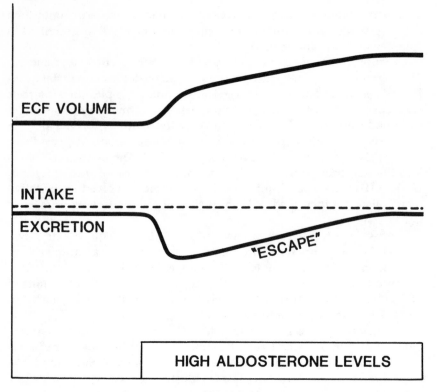

DAYS

Figure 9-9.   The phenomenon of "mineralocorticoid escape" and its effect on extra-cellular fluid volume.

nerve at levels below that required to alter RPF or GFR increases salt and water reabsorption in the proximal tubule. The significance of this effect in mediating the renal response to alterations in ECF volume is not yet known.

ADH

Severe volume depletion has been shown to be a potent stimulus for ADH secretion. A drop in blood volume of 15 to 20% can elevate ADH blood levels to a point more than twice that of the most effective osmotic stimulus. This response is believed to be triggered by stimuli sensed by left atrial and arterial baroreceptors.

Figure 9-10 compares the changes in ADH secretion that occur in response to changes in ECF osmotic concentration and volume. The changes in osmotic concentration were made without altering volume and vice versa. It is clear that the release of ADH by the pituitary is much more sensitive to osmotic concentration changes. A rise in ADH plasma levels in response to volume depletion is not apparent until a 10% decrease in volume occurs, whereas a 1% increase in osmotic concentration causes a discernable change in ADH release.

There is a more subtle interrelationship between osmotic and volume stimuli than is apparent in Figure 9-10. A decrease in blood volume has been shown to reduce the threshold osmotic concentration at which ADH secretion can be triggered and to increase the sensitivity of the osmoreceptors to osmotic stimuli. A hypothetical model has been devel-

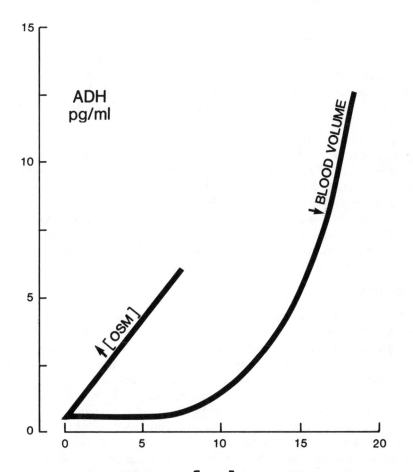

PERCENT CHANGE IN [OSM] OR BLOOD VOLUME

Figure 9-10. The relative effects of an increase in extracellular fluid osmolality, and a decrease in blood volume on the plasma concentration of ADH. (Adapted from a figure in: Dunn, F. L., Brennan, T. J., Nelson, A. E., and Robertson, G. L.: The role of blood osmolality and volume in regulating vasopressin secretion in the rat. J. Clin. Invest., 52:3212, 1973.)

oped to describe this interrelationship. The model proposes that the neurosecretory cells for ADH receive input from two populations of neurons. One is activated by osmoreceptors and the other by volume receptors. According to this model, decreased input from volume receptors during volume depletion may sensitize the neurosecretory cells to input from osmoreceptors.

As indicated in Figure 9-10, volume depletion can raise plasma ADH concentrations much above that required to induce maximum antidiuresis (4.5 to 5.0 pg/ml, Fig. 9-3). The physiologic "usefulness" of the excess ADH is not clear, but probably is related to its known vasoconstrictor properties.

Natriuretic Hormone

It is possible that a natriuretic or "salt-losing" hormone may exist. An unknown substance is present in the urine of volume-expanded animals that depresses salt transport by a variety of epithelia. However, the nature of the substance, its site of origin, and the factors that control its release are unknown.

In severe renal disease, when the functioning nephron population is greatly reduced and uremia occurs, the remaining nephrons increase their excretion of salt and water tremendously and the body is still able to regulate its ECF volume. There are strong indications that a humoral factor is responsible for the inhibition of reabsorption in these nephrons. It is not yet clear whether this humoral factor is a physiologic substance that accumulates in abnormal amounts during this disease or an abnormal product of the deranged metabolism that is characteristic of this disease.

SUMMARY

Extracellular fluid volume is regulated by a variety of receptors and overlapping effector mechanisms. Our knowledge regarding the receptors and the mechanisms they activate is fragmentary. Furthermore, we are uncertain of the role each receptor and each mechanism plays in the various types of ECF fluid volume disturbance. Nevertheless, it is useful to attempt to piece together the fragments of our knowledge. Figures 9-11 and 9-12 are attempts to do so by showing the response to severe volume depletion and to acute volume expansion.

In severe volume depletion, there are two triggering stimuli: the fall in arterial pressure and the fall in venous volume (Fig. 9-11). These stimuli activate two major systems, the sympathetic nervous system and the juxtaglomerular apparatus. These two systems are interrelated in that the sympathetic nervous system also stimulates the juxtaglomerular apparatus. As a result, the activity of the renin-angiotensin-aldosterone axis is increased. This, plus a constellation of other effector mech-

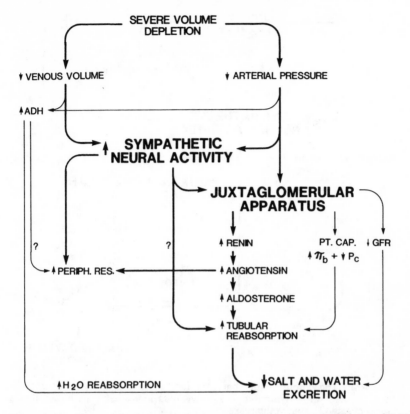

Figure 9-11. The various factors that respond to severe volume depletion and act to reduce the excretion of salt and water. In mild volume depletion, the pathways indicated by the heavy lines are probably the primary ones activated.

anisms, reduces the excretion of salt and water. In addition, total peripheral resistance is raised by the sympathetic neural and humoral activity in combination with angiotensin, so that the effect of the loss of circulating blood volume is minimized. The sympathetic nervous system also decreases venous compliance and increases the pumping activity of the heart. In mild volume depletion, not all the effector mechanisms shown in the figure would be activated. It is probable that the pathways indicated by the heavy arrows would prevail in that situation.

The response to acute expansion of ECF volume induced by infusion of saline has been studied extensively in experimental animals. This may occur only rarely in humans. Nevertheless, it provides a useful framework for summarizing our knowledge of the response to increased ECF volume (Fig. 9-12). Again, the sympathetic nervous system and juxtaglomerular apparatus are the two major systems that respond. The

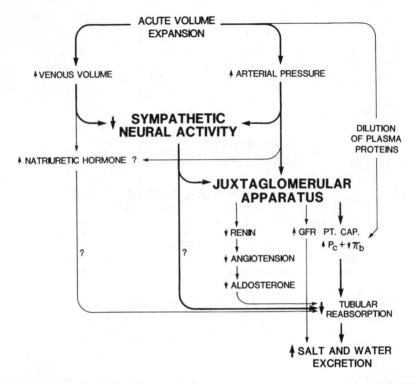

Figure 9-12. The various factors that respond to acute volume expansion and act to increase salt and water excretion. The heavy lines indicate the pathways that are probably activated in mild volume expansion.

change in peritubular capillary pressures is probably the major cause of the resulting diuresis. The fall in π_b in the peritubular capillary may be accentuated by dilution of plasma protein concentration by the infused fluid. Presumably, the activity of natriuretic hormone, if it exists, would also be increased. In the acute response to volume expansion, the renin-angiotensin-aldosterone axis is unimportant. In the chronic situation, the reduced levels of aldosterone are an important factor in causing increased excretion of salt and water.

BIBLIOGRAPHY

General:

Andreoli, T. E., Grantham, J. J., and Rector, F. C. Jr. (Eds.): Disturbances in Body Fluid Osmolality. Bethesda, American Physiological Society, 1977.
See the following chapters from: Brenner, B. M. and Rector, F. C. Jr., (Eds.): The Kidney. 2nd ed. Philadelphia, W. B. Saunders Co., 1981.
    Chapter 7. Burg, M. B.: Renal Handling of Sodium Chloride, Water, Amino Acids and Glucose.

Chapter 8. Seely, J. F., and Levy, M.: Control of Extracellular Fluid Volume.
Chapter 15. Levy, M., and Seely, J. F.: Pathophysiology of Edema Formation.
Chapter 16. Hays, R. M., and Levine, S. D.: Pathophysiology of Water Metabolism.
Reineck, H. J., and Stein, J. H.: Renal Regulation of Extracellular Fluid Volume. *In* Sodium
and Water Homeostasis. Edited by B. M. Brenner, and J. H. Stein, Contemporary Issues
in Nephrology. Vol. 1. New York, Churchill Livingstone, 1978.
Skorecki, K. L., and Brenner, B. M.: Body fluid homeostasis in man. Am. J. Med., *70*:77,
1981.
Stein, J. H., Lameire, N. H., and Earley, L. E.: Renal Hemodynamic Factors and the
Regulation of Sodium Excretion. *In* Physiology of Membrane Disorders. Edited by T. E.
Andreoli, J. F. Hoffman, and D. D. Fanestil. New York, Plenum Medical Book Co.,1978.

Specific:

Davis, J. O., and Freeman, R. H.: Mechanisms regulating renin release. Physiol. Rev.,
56:1, 1976.
Dibona, G. F.: Neurogenic regulation of renal tubular sodium reabsorption. Am. J.
Physiol., *233* (Renal Fluid Electrolyte Physiol. 2):F73, 1977.
Dousa, T. P., and Valtin, H.: Cellular actions of vasopressin in the mammalian kidney.
Kidney Internat., *10*:46, 1976.
Fanestil, D. D., and Park, C. S.: Steroid hormones and the kidney. Ann. Rev. Physiol.,
43:637, 1981.
Goetz, K. L., Bond, G. C., and Bloxham, D. D.: Atrial receptors and renal function.
Physiol. Rev., *55*:157,1975.
Gottschalk, C. W.: Renal nerves and sodium excretion. Ann. Rev. Physiol., *43*:229, 1981.
Handler, J. S., and Orloff, J.: Antidiuretic hormone. Ann. Rev. Physiol., *43*:611, 1981.
Reid, I. A., Morris, B. J., and Ganong, W. F.: The renin-angiotensin system. Ann. Rev.
Physiol., *40*:377, 1978.
Robertson, G. L., Shelton, R. L., and Athar, S.: The osmoregulation of vasopressin.
Kidney Internat., *10*:25, 1976.
Schrier, R. W., Berl, T., and Anderson, R. J.: Osmotic and nonosmotic control of vaso-
pressin release. Am. J. Physiol., *236* (Renal Fluid Electrolyte Physiol. 5):F321, 1979.

CHAPTER *10*

The Role of the Kidney in Acid-Base Regulation

The kidney plays a primary role in the complex process that maintains a constant hydrogen ion activity in body fluids. Figure 10-1 presents a simplified diagram of this process. The figure depicts the buffer systems in blood; how these buffer systems react to acid and alkali produced by tissue metabolism; and the interrelationships among these buffering systems, the excretion of acid and alkali by the kidney and the excretion of CO_2 by the lungs. CO_2 produced by metabolic processes in body tissue reacts with water to form H_2CO_3, which dissociates to H^+ and HCO_3^- (Reaction 1). This hydration of CO_2 is catalyzed by the enzyme carbonic anhydrase, which is present in red blood cells. Hydrogen ions produced by that reaction combine with hemoglobin and other buffers in the blood (Reaction 2). Other acids and alkalis produced by cellular metabolism are also buffered by these two systems. These two buffer systems are in dynamic equilibrium with the same hydrogen ion concentration (pH), so that a change induced in the concentration of any one factor in either reaction rapidly affects the other reaction and a new hydrogen ion concentration in the blood is established.

The lungs assist in maintaining a constant blood pH by removing CO_2, while the kidney excretes acid in the form of H_2PO_4 and NH_4 and alkali in the form of HCO_3. The buffer systems in blood and the actions of the lungs and kidneys maintain the P_{CO_2} (partial pressure of CO_2) at 40 mm Hg, the hydrogen ion concentration at about 40 nanoequivalents/liter (10^{-9} Eq/L, pH = 7.4) and the bicarbonate concentration at about 25 milliequivalents/liter (mEq/L).

The kidney contributes to the regulation of acid-base balance in two ways. First, it corrects disturbances that result from imbalanced food intake or internal metabolic disorders. Normally, in members of a population whose diet contains a significant amount of animal protein, cellular metabolism results in net addition of acid to the blood, approximately 1 mEq/kg body weight per day. The kidney responds to this by

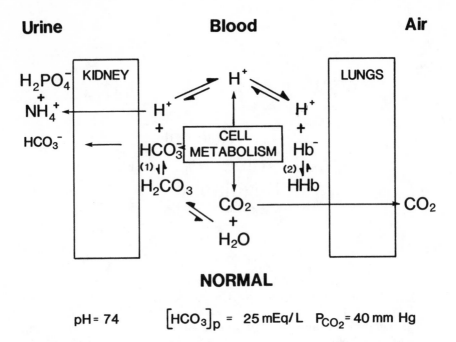

NORMAL

$pH = 74$ $[HCO_3]_p = 25\,mEq/L$ $P_{CO_2} = 40\,mm\,Hg$

Figure 10-1. The acid-base buffering systems of the body. The arrows across the box representing the kidney indicate excretion only. They are not meant to convey any information on the renal mechanisms involved.

forming and extracting an acid fluid from the blood. Secondly, the kidney compensates for acid-base imbalances that result when respiratory disorders alter the rate of ventilation of the lung and subsequently the P_{CO_2} of tissue fluids.

Whatever the nature of the disturbance, the response of the kidney leads to the formation and extraction from the plasma of a fluid with an excess or a deficit of acid. The primary result is a return of the H ion concentration of the blood toward the normal level.

The primary renal mechanism involved in acid-base control is the process that secretes H ions into the tubular fluid. The buffer systems in tubular fluid that react with the secreted H ions are similar in many ways to those in blood. The buffer pair $HCO_3 : H_2CO_3$ is as important in tubular fluid as it is in blood. There is also a nonbicarbonate buffering system as in blood, except that hemoglobin and other proteins are not included among these buffers. The lungs perform the same function of controlling the P_{CO_2} of tubular cells and tubular fluid as they do of other cells and fluids in the body. There is one unique feature: the tubular cells produce a buffer, ammonia. The concentration of ammonia in urine and, thus, its contribution to the buffering of secreted H ions increase as the urine becomes more acid.

HYDROGEN ION SECRETION

Within tubular cells, enzymatic processes generate hydrogen ions and hydroxyl ions from water in spatially separated loci. The hydrogen ions are secreted into the tubular lumen (Fig. 10-2). The resulting increase in hydroxyl ions within the cell is buffered by H ions obtained from the hydration of CO_2 and the subsequent ionization of H_2CO_3. The HCO_3 created in that hydration leaves the cell and enters the interstitial fluid. The enzyme carbonic anhydrase catalyzes the reaction between H_2O and CO_2.

An active transport process located in the luminal membrane is responsible for the secretion of H ions. The exact nature of this mechanism is not known. It may be a primary transport process that transports net charge in the form of protons into the tubular lumen. If this occurs, the secretion probably is electrically balanced by diffusion of Na from the tubular fluid into the cell. It is also possible that it is a secondary active process, an "antiport," which exchanges H for Na in a tightly coupled manner. The energy for this process could be supplied by the electrochemical gradient for Na established by the activity of Na-K-ATPase. With either type of system, the net result is the same: the exchange of

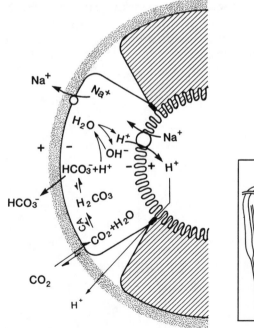
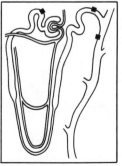

Figure 10-2. The mechanism of H^+ secretion by tubular cells. The ion may be secreted by an antiport mechanism located in the apical membrane which exchanges H^+ in the cell for Na in the tubular fluid. CA = carbonic anhydrase.

H^+ for Na^+. The HCO_3 generated within the cell is considered to move passively into the interstitial fluid down an electrochemical gradient.

The H ion transport system is gradient-limited. In other words, the active flux into the lumen is countered by a passive leak or back-flux out of the tubule. Evidently, the various sections of the nephron differ in their conductance to H in somewhat the same manner as in their conductance to Na. In the proximal tubule, the limiting concentration gradient, at which the active flux of H into the lumen is balanced by the passive flux out, is reached at a tubular fluid pH of about 6.8 in the rat and about 7.1 in the dog. In the rat the distal tubular value is 6.4. The collecting duct can set up and maintain the largest gradient. In man, the urine leaving the collecting ducts may have a pH as low as 4.5. This corresponds to a concentration gradient of about 800:1.

Two major factors determine the extent of H ion secretion: the tubular fluid buffer concentration and the Pco_2 of arterial blood (Fig. 10-3). Buffers present in the tubular fluid remove secreted H ions from solution, thereby maintaining a high pH in tubular fluid. This permits more H ions to be secreted before the limiting concentration gradient is reached. Bicarbonate is the most abundant buffer in the glomerular filtrate and factors that alter its concentration in tubular fluid strongly affect the rate of H secretion. Water reabsorption tends to maintain the bicarbonate concentration high and this permits a high rate of secretion. Inhibition of fluid reabsorption, particularly in the proximal tubule, causes the bicarbonate concentration to drop rapidly as it is titrated by secreted H. Thus, the limiting concentration gradient is rapidly reached and net secretion is reduced. If the inhibition of fluid reabsorption is

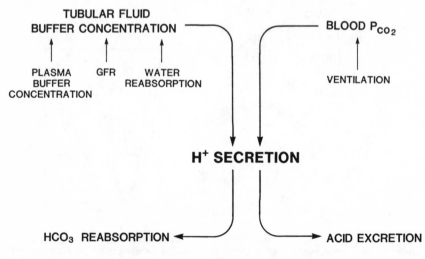

Figure 10-3. The factors controlling the rate of hydrogen secretion.

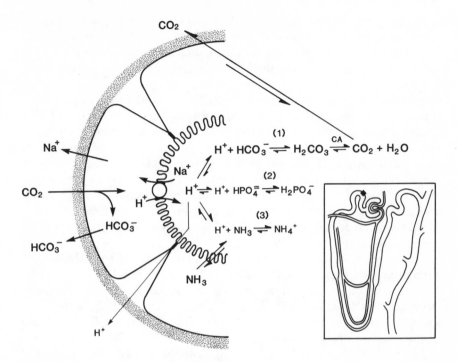

Figure 10-4. Tubular fluid buffer reactions in the proximal tubule. Reaction 1 predominates here.

due to ECF volume expansion, it is possible that the paracellular conductance to ions including H is increased (Chapter 9). The resulting rise in passive back-flux of H would further limit net secretion. Changes in GFR alter the amount of bicarbonate filtered per unit time, and therefore, alter the amount of H ions required to reduce the buffer concentration. The rate of H secretion is also affected by the P_{CO_2}, which evidently regulates the supply of H ions to the transport mechanism. This factor is probably more important in chronic acid-base imbalances than in acute disturbances.

BUFFER REACTIONS WITHIN THE TUBULAR FLUID

When H ions enter the tubule, they combine with the various buffers present in the tubular fluid. As indicated in Reaction 1 in Figure 10-4, secreted H ions may combine with filtered HCO_3 to form H_2O and CO_2. In the process, one HCO_3 ion disappears from the tubular fluid and one HCO_3 ion appears in the peritubular plasma. The CO_2 that is formed diffuses out of the tubule. The net result is the reabsorption of Na and HCO_3, a slight fall in urine pH, and no change in the P_{CO_2} of the tubular fluid.

In the proximal tubule, but not elsewhere, carbonic anhydrase is attached to the cell membranes and is in contact with the tubular fluid. By catalyzing the dehydration of H_2CO_3, it facilitates the reabsorption of HCO_3 and helps to prevent the H ion concentration from increasing to a point that would reduce the net secretion of the ion.

Secreted H ions also combine with $HPO_4^=$ and other fixed buffer anions (Reaction 2 in Fig. 10-4). The net result is the extraction of acid from the ECF and the reabsorption of Na. Phosphate is one of the more important urinary buffers; its pK is 6.8, close to the pH of the filtrate, and acceptance of H still leaves it with one negative charge. Thus, it remains lipid-insoluble and cannot diffuse back into blood carrying H with it. Other buffer anions present in smaller amounts are also titrated in the same fashion. One of these is creatinine. In uncontrolled diabetes mellitus, β-hydroxybutyric acid and acetoacetic acid are important urine buffers.

As shown in Reaction 3 in Figure 10-4, H ions may also combine with ammonia. Uncharged, lipid-soluble NH_3, produced from glutamine within the tubular cell, diffuses into the urine. Secreted H ions combine with NH_3 to form charged, lipid-insoluble NH_4^+, which is then excreted. The net result is the extraction of acid from the ECF and the reabsorption of Na.

For reasons that will be described, Reaction 1 predominates in the proximal tubule as illustrated in Figure 10-4. In the distal sections of the nephron, the bicarbonate concentration in tubular fluid is usually low, and Reactions 2 and 3 occur to a greater extent (Fig. 10-5).

THE ISOHYDRIC PRINCIPLE

The extent to which each of the reactions in Figures 10-4 and 10-5 occurs depends on the isohydric principle. In the reaction of any buffer with hydrogen ion $H^+ + A^- \rightleftarrows HA$, the ratio of the concentration of the two forms, [HA]/[A], is determined by the concentration of H in the solution and the dissociation constant, K, for the reaction. The isohydric principle states that all buffers in a common solution must be in equilibrium with the same H concentration. The isohydric principle is expressed by the following equation:

$$[H] = \frac{[HA_1]}{[A_1]} K_1 = \frac{[HA_2]}{[A_2]} K_2 = \frac{[HA_3]}{[A_3]} K_3$$

Considering the three most important buffers in tubular fluid and changing the equation to its log form:

$$pH = pK_1 + \log \frac{[HCO_3]}{S \cdot P_{CO_2}} = pK_2 + \log \frac{[HPO_4]}{[H_2PO_4]} = pK_3 + \log \frac{[NH_3]}{[NH_4]}$$

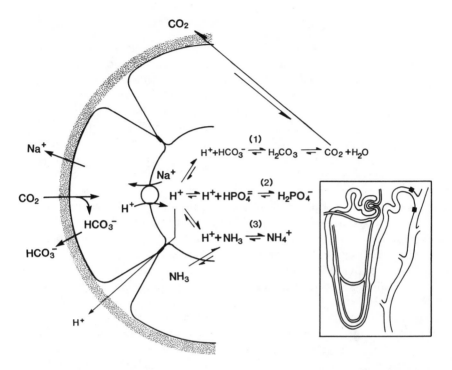

Figure 10-5. Tubular fluid buffer reactions in the distal tubule and collecting duct. Reactions 2 and 3 usually predominate here.

S is the solubility coefficient for CO_2 and the term $S \cdot P_{CO_2}$ then is the concentration of dissolved CO_2 and H_2CO_3 in solution. The value of S for plasma is 0.03. pK_1, pK_2, pK_3 are the specific pKs for each buffer pair.

The isohydric equation tells us the following. As H ions are added to the tubular fluid, some of each of the buffers will be titrated to the acidic form. The extent to which each is titrated depends on: (1) the amount of H ions secreted; (2) the concentration of each buffer present (if a large concentration of one buffer is present in its basic form, it takes more H ions to shift the ratio [A]/[HA] significantly and titration of other buffers is reduced accordingly); and (3) the pK of the individual buffer. Those buffers with a pK close to the pH of the filtrate will be titrated to a much greater extent than those with a pK far removed from that level. The pKs of each of the major urine buffers are approximately:

$$HCO_3/S \cdot P_{CO_2} : pK = 6.1$$

$$HPO_4/H_2PO_4 : pK = 6.8$$

$$NH_3/NH_4 : pK = 9.0$$

BICARBONATE REABSORPTION

The buffer pair $HCO_3/S \cdot Pco_2$ is an important urinary buffer despite its low pK for two reasons. First, the concentration of HCO_3 in the filtrate is greater than the concentration of any other buffer. Second, the kidney can alter only the concentration of the alkaline member of the buffer pair. It has little control over the concentration of the acid form, since the tubular epithelium is permeable to CO_2. Thus, the reabsorption of water from the filtrate tends to make the urine alkaline, because the concentration of only the alkaline form of this buffer will rise. H secretion lowers the concentration of the alkaline form, but causes only a limited increase in the concentration of the acid form, because CO_2 diffuses out of the tubular fluid as it is generated. The lungs, by controlling the Pco_2 of blood, also control the Pco_2 of tubular fluid and thereby exert an influence on tubular fluid pH and on all acid-base reactions that are influenced by the pH. For these reasons, HCO_3 reabsorption accounts for over 90% of the mass of H ions secreted. Thus a description of the kidneys' reaction to acid-base disturbances must begin with an account of bicarbonate reabsorption and excretion.

The factors affecting bicarbonate reabsorption and excretion are shown in Figure 10-6. The primary factor is the plasma bicarbonate concentration, which determines the concentration in the glomerular filtrate entering the tubule. Net H ion secretion and bicarbonate reabsorption from the tubular fluid continue until the H ion concentration

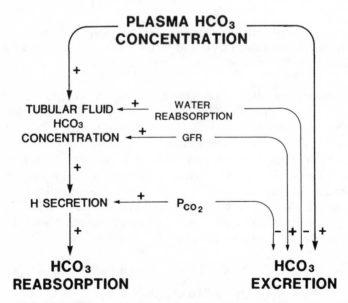

Figure 10-6. The factors controlling the rates of bicarbonate reabsorption and excretion.

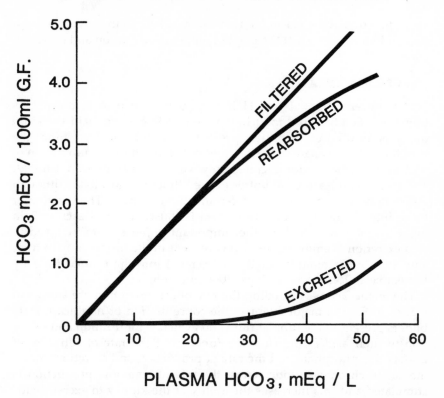

Figure 10-7. The quantitative relationship between the plasma bicarbonate concentration and the rates of filtration, reabsorption, and excretion of bicarbonate. G.F. = glomerular filtrate.

rises (and bicarbonate concentration falls) to the point at which the limiting gradient for net secretion is reached. Water reabsorption tends to increase the bicarbonate concentration without altering the concentration of the acid form of the buffer pair, so tubular fluid pH rises. Thus, additional H secretion and bicarbonate reabsorption can occur. GFR also affects bicarbonate reabsorption and excretion by altering the mass of bicarbonate filtered per unit time. The blood P_{CO_2} influences the rate of bicarbonate reabsorption by affecting the rate of H secretion.

Figure 10-7 illustrates the quantitative relationship between the plasma bicarbonate concentration and the rates of reabsorption and excretion. When the plasma concentration is below the normal level of 25 mEq/L, almost all the filtered bicarbonate is reabsorbed; the rate of excretion is low. When the bicarbonate concentration rises above normal, reabsorption increases. However, not all the increment in filtered bicarbonate is reabsorbed, so the excretion of bicarbonate also rises. Thus, both the rates of reabsorption *and* excretion change in the same direction as the plasma concentration. Changes in water reabsorption and blood P_{CO_2} shift the position of the reabsorption and excretion curves.

EXCRETION OF ACID

The concentration of free H ions in urine, even at a low pH, is minimal (pH 4.5 = .032 mEq/L), so the effectiveness of acid excretion depends on titration of buffers present in the tubular fluid. Since the titration of bicarbonate to H_2CO_3 does not result in the accumulation of acid in the urine, acid is excreted only when other buffers are titrated. The major nonbicarbonate buffer in the filtrate is phosphate, although others may be of importance in certain circumstances. The titration of these filtered, nonbicarbonate buffers is illustrated by Reaction 2 in Figures 10-4 and 10-5. The other important buffer system involved in acid excretion is ammonia, which is present in the filtrate only in trace amounts, but is manufactured and secreted into the tubular fluid by tubular cells (Reaction 3 in Figs. 10-4 and 10-5).

The major factors controlling the rate of acid excretion are shown in Figure 10-8. One major factor is the concentration of nonbicarbonate buffers present in the tubular fluid and available for titration and excretion in their acid form. This is a function of the rate of filtration of buffers like phosphate and the rate of production and secretion of ammonia. In chronic acidotic states, the rate of ammonia production is stimulated and this increases the ability of the kidney to excrete acid.

As the isohydric principle indicates, the titration and excretion of the nonbicarbonate buffers in their acid form is favored when the tubular fluid hydrogen concentration is high (pH is low). The two major factors affecting this concentration are the plasma HCO_3 concentration and the blood P_{CO_2}. When the HCO_3 concentration in the plasma and thus in the filtrate is high, Reaction 1 in Figure 10-4 goes to the right, but H_2CO_3 does not accumulate and the H concentration of tubular fluid is kept low (pH high), slowing Reactions 2 and 3. For this reason, bicarbonate reabsorption predominates in the proximal tubule and only small amounts of acid are titrated (Fig. 10-4). When the bicarbonate concentration falls, Reaction 1 slows, the tubular fluid H concentration rises, and Reactions 2 and 3 proceed at a greater rate. In the tubular fluid reaching the distal tubule, the bicarbonate concentration is usually, but not always, low and, as H is secreted, Reactions 2 and 3 can take place at a faster rate than in the proximal tubule (Fig. 10-5).

When the blood P_{CO_2} is elevated, H secretion increases, at least in chronic states. This tends to increase the concentration in tubular fluid and Reactions 2 and 3 are driven to the right. There is an additional effect of a rise in P_{CO_2}. Since the tubular epithelium is highly permeable to CO_2, the tubular fluid P_{CO_2} always changes in response to changes in blood P_{CO_2}. A rise in tubular fluid P_{CO_2} increases the concentration of

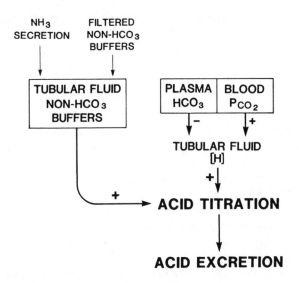

Figure 10-8. The factors regulating the rates of acid titration and excretion.

H_2CO_3 and thus the H concentration. This also increases acid titration.

The quantitative effect of changes in the bicarbonate concentration and P_{CO_2} of tubular fluid are illustrated in the following examples. Consider that a rise in the plasma bicarbonate concentration increases the rate of HCO_3 excretion, and its concentration in the final urine rises from 5 to 10 mEq/L. If there is no change in P_{CO_2}, the buffer equation indicates the urine pH would rise:

$$pH = 6.1 + \log \frac{5}{0.03 \times 40} = 6.72$$

$$pH = 6.1 + \log \frac{10}{0.03 \times 40} = 7.02$$

The isohydric principle indicates that the rise in pH would reduce the titration of phosphate and ammonia, and thus the rate of acid excretion would fall. If hypoventilation raises the blood P_{CO_2} and thence the urine P_{CO_2} from 40 to 60 mm Hg and if the urine bicarbonate concentration is maintained at 5 mEq/L, the buffer equation indicates that the urine pH would fall from 6.72 to 6.54. According to the isohydric principle, titration of phosphate and NH_3 to their acid form would increase, and thus the rate of acid excretion would be greater.

It should be realized that the P_{CO_2} of the final urine may not be exactly equal to that of blood. It is often higher, and on rare occasions, may be lower. Higher values are perhaps due to countercurrent trapping of CO_2

and also to delayed dehydration of H_2CO_3 formed in distal sections of the nephron. Nevertheless, the major factor controlling the tubular fluid P_{CO_2} is the blood P_{CO_2}, which in turn, is controlled by pulmonary ventilation.

CONTRIBUTION OF THE NEPHRON SEGMENTS

Among the nephron segments, the proximal tubule has the greatest capacity to secrete H, but the high permeability of the epithelium allows it to establish and maintain only a limited transepithelial concentration gradient. Thus, it is able to reabsorb a large fraction of the filtered bicarbonate (>75%), but it can reduce the tubular fluid pH only to a slight extent, and therefore, titrates relatively small amounts of the other buffers (Fig. 10-4). It may be classed as a high capacity—low gradient system. The inability to establish a large gradient also causes it to pass on increased amounts of bicarbonate to the distal segments whenever water reabsorption is reduced.

Bicarbonate is reabsorbed in the loop of Henle pari passu with water, so that the concentration of bicarbonate and the pH of the tubular fluid entering the distal tubule (8 mEq/L HCO_3 and pH 6.7, in the rat) is close to that leaving the proximal tubule.

The hydrogen secretory mechanism in the distal and collecting tubules, in contrast to that in the proximal tubule, has a low capacity but is capable of generating a high transepithelial gradient. The tubular fluid delivered to these segments normally has a bicarbonate concentration much lower than that in the filtrate, and thus the low capacity of the hydrogen secretory mechanism is not devoted entirely to bicarbonate titration. The relative impermeability of the epithelium enables the secretory mechanism to raise the H ion concentration of tubular fluid and effectively titrate phosphate and ammonia to their acid forms (Fig. 10-5). Normally, therefore, bicarbonate reabsorption occurs primarily in the proximal tubule (Fig. 10-4) and acid titration occurs primarily in the distal segments (Fig. 10-5).

If bicarbonate reabsorption is reduced in the proximal tubule and delivery to the distal segments is increased, the rate of bicarbonate reabsorption in the distal segments will increase and titration of nonbicarbonate buffers will be slowed. However, the low capacity of the distal mechanism can often be swamped by the overload of bicarbonate, so that bicarbonate excretion will increase.

Failure of either the proximal (high capacity—low gradient) or the distal (low capacity—high gradient) secretory mechanism is seen in several clinical states. Failure of the proximal mechanism causes acidosis (proximal renal tubular acidosis) because more bicarbonate is passed on to the low capacity distal mechanism than it can reabsorb. The loss of alkali in the urine causes the body fluids to become acidotic. In these patients, the urine pH can still be reduced to a minimal level

(<pH 5.0) by decreasing the filtered load of bicarbonate to the point that the unaffected distal mechanism can reabsorb the excess bicarbonate leaving the proximal tubule. A defect in the distal mechanism (distal renal tubular acidosis) can be recognized by the inability of the kidney to reduce urine pH below 5.0, even when the filtered load of bicarbonate is reduced.

RENAL REACTION TO ACID-BASE IMBALANCES

To reiterate, the kidney responds to acid-base imbalances by forming and extracting from the ECF a fluid that contains an excess of acid or alkali. The net effect is a return of blood pH towards the normal value of 7.4. In metabolic acid-base derangements, this also leads to a return of the plasma bicarbonate concentration towards the normal level of 25 mEq/L. In respiratory disorders however, the renal response maintains the blood pH near 7.4 but drives the plasma bicarbonate above or below the normal level.

The two major factors that govern the kidneys' response to acid-base disorders are the plasma bicarbonate concentration and the blood P_{CO_2}. The plasma bicarbonate concentration is the major factor that alters the rate of bicarbonate excretion (Figs. 10-6 and 10-7) and one of the three major factors that controls the rate of acid excretion (Fig. 10-8). The blood P_{CO_2} is also one of the three major factors controlling the rate of acid excretion. The third factor involved in controlling acid excretion, the buffer concentration of tubular fluid, affects the degree but not the direction of the renal response.

Response to Respiratory Disorders

Consider first the response to respiratory acidosis. Figure 10-9a illustrates the type of changes that occur in the body. An acute reduction in the ventilation of the lungs causes the P_{CO_2} of the blood to rise. This drives Reaction 1 to increase the concentration of HCO_3 and H. The H ions are buffered by hemoglobin and other blood and tissue buffers. Because of this buffering, the H concentration of blood increases by only a few nanoequivalents while the increase in bicarbonate is in the milliequivalent range. Representative values for pH, plasma bicarbonate concentration, and P_{CO_2} in acute respiratory acidosis are listed in the figure. These are typical of values that would exist before renal compensation begins.

The kidney responds to this situation by increasing the excretion of acid. Figure 10-10 indicates how this comes about. The rise in P_{CO_2} increases the concentration of H ions in tubular fluid and with time stimulates H secretion. This causes the titration of HPO_4 and NH_3 to proceed at a faster rate. If the primary respiratory disorder persists for 2 to 3 days, the rate of ammonia production by tubular cells also rises. These factors combine to increase the rate of acid titration and excretion.

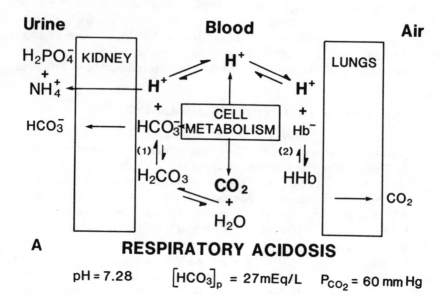

A **RESPIRATORY ACIDOSIS**

$pH = 7.28$ $\left[HCO_3\right]_p = 27 mEq/L$ $P_{CO_2} = 60\,mm\,Hg$

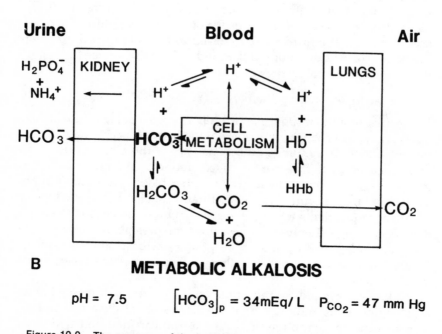

B **METABOLIC ALKALOSIS**

$pH = 7.5$ $\left[HCO_3\right]_p = 34 mEq/L$ $P_{CO_2} = 47\,mm\,Hg$

Figure 10-9. The response of the buffering systems of the body to (A) respiratory acidosis caused by hypoventilation of the lungs and (B) metabolic alkalosis.

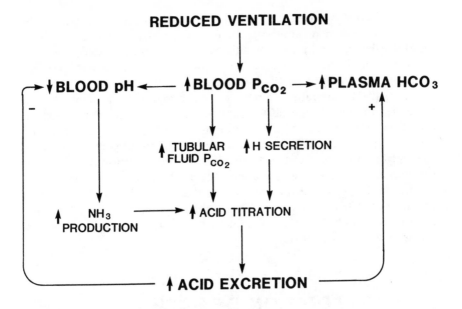

Figure 10-10. The factors governing the response of the kidney to respiratory acidosis.

The continual removal by the kidney of hydrogen ions from the blood reduces the H ion concentration (raises blood pH) and drives Reaction 1 in Figure 10-9 so that the HCO_3 concentration of plasma increases still further. Reaction 2 is also affected, so that the concentration of the basic form of hemoglobin and other buffers returns toward the normal level. In patients with chronic obstructive lung disease, the compensation for the acidosis increases with time. That is to say, the kidneys increase the rate of acid removal from blood, and the blood pH returns almost to normal. This means that in a patient maintaining a blood Pco_2 of 60 mm Hg, the plasma bicarbonate concentration rises to 34 to 36 mEq/L. Over 80% of the compensation for the acidosis is due to the response of the kidney. Less than 20% is due to chemical buffering by the blood and body tissue.

Response to Metabolic Disorders

Figure 10-9b illustrates how the body reacts to metabolic alkalosis. This condition can result, for instance, from chronic ingestion of antacids or from chronic loss of gastric secretions by vomiting. Either results in the net addition of alkali to the blood by the gastrointestinal system. The bicarbonate concentration in blood rises and combines with H to form CO_2 and H_2O. The drop in the H ion concentration of blood is partly counteracted by increased dissociation of HHb. The respiratory system responds to the fall in the H ion concentration by hypoventilating the lungs. The subsequent rise in P_{CO_2} partly compensates for the alkalosis. Typical values for metabolic alkalosis, partially compensated by hypoventilation, are listed in the figure.

Figure 10-11 illustrates the renal response to metabolic alkalosis. The large rise in the plasma HCO_3 concentration increases the rate of its excretion (Figs. 10-6 and 10-7). The rise in the tubular fluid concentration of bicarbonate, particularly in the distal tubule, reduces the H concentration of the fluid and this reverses the direction of phosphate titration and reduces the formation of NH_4. This is partly counteracted by the rise in P_{CO_2}, but the net effect is that an alkaline fluid is formed and extracted from the blood. This serves to correct the alkalosis and return the blood back to a normal hydrogen ion activity and normal bicarbonate concentration.

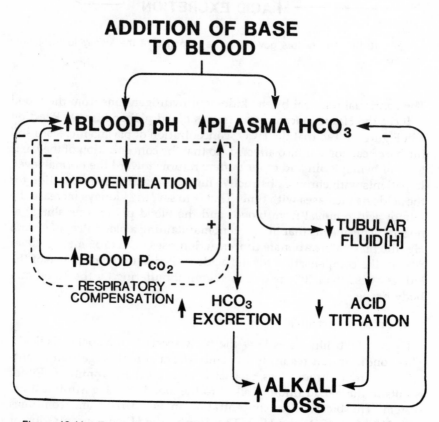

Figure 10-11. The factors governing the response of the kidney to metabolic alkalosis.

The patterns the kidney follows in response to respiratory alkalosis and metabolic acidosis can be discerned from the foregoing discussion. It is important to note that the result of the renal response to respiratory disturbances of acid-base balance differs fundamentally from the response to metabolic disturbances. The former is a *compensation*, blood pH is returned toward the normal point but the plasma bicarbonate concentration is driven away from the normal level. The latter is a *correction*, both the pH and the plasma bicarbonate concentration are returned to the normal level.

THE ROLE OF CARBONIC ANHYDRASE

The enzyme carbonic anhydrase plays a key role in the kidneys' response to acid-base disturbances. The enzyme catalyzes the reaction $H_2O + CO_2 \rightleftarrows H_2CO_3$ in either direction, increasing the rate of the reaction by a factor of 10^4. The law of mass action determines the direction the reaction will take. Within tubular cells, the activity of the enzyme tends to maintain cell pH constant. It does so by providing H ions to balance the alkali released within the cell by the hydrogen secretory mechanism. Inhibition of the enzyme's activity may cause cell pH to rise and retard the secretion of H ions.

The enzyme is also present on the tubular surface of proximal tubular cells and is in contact with the tubular fluid. Its activity there speeds the process of bicarbonate reabsorption and thus increases the rate of the entire process of salt and water reabsorption. To be more specific, H ions secreted into the tubular lumen combine with HCO_3 to form H_2CO_3. The enzyme catalyzes the dehydration of the acid to H_2O and CO_2. The loss of anion HCO_3^- from the tubular fluid promotes the reabsorption of cations, predominantly Na^+. This removal of solute particles from the tubular fluid increases the osmotic reabsorption of water. Inhibition of carbonic anhydrase reduces the rate of dehydration of H_2CO_3. Bicarbonate reabsorption is reduced, and this, in turn, slows down Na and water reabsorption.

Compounds that contain an unsubstituted SO_2NH_2 group may inhibit carbonic anhydrase. By so doing, they reduce the rate of H secretion and slow the rate of bicarbonate reabsorption. Na and water reabsorption are then reduced. Such compounds were, at one time, used clinically to cause diuresis, the loss of salt and water. Examples of such drugs are acetazolamide and dichlorphenamide. Other diuretic agents such as those of the thiazide group (chlorothiazide, bendroflumethiazide, and the like) also possess the ability to inhibit carbonic anhydrase to varying degrees, although this is not the major mechanism by which they cause diuresis.

Inhibition of carbonic anhydrase causes the kidney to form and extract an alkaline fluid from the blood resulting in acidemia. This is one of the main side effects of diuretic agents that primarily inhibit carbonic anhydrase. They also increase K excretion and thus can cause hypokalemia (see Chapter 11).

RELATIONSHIP TO SALT AND WATER REABSORPTION

Several factors contribute to a close interdependence between the renal mechanisms involved in regulating acid-base balance and those responsible for maintenance of salt and water balance. Bicarbonate represents over 17% of the anions accompanying Na in the filtrate, and thus, alterations in the reabsorption of one can easily affect reabsorption of the other. Changes in the reabsorption of either ion also affect the reabsorption of water. A good example of this is the effect of carbonic anhydrase inhibitors on bicarbonate, sodium, and water reabsorption in the proximal tubule as has been described.

On the other hand, alterations in GFR and in fluid reabsorption in the proximal tubule can greatly alter the rate of bicarbonate reabsorption (Fig. 10-6). In addition, the effect of aldosterone on cells of the collecting tubule enhances their ability to secrete hydrogen. When ECF volume is expanded, the resulting reduction in fluid reabsorption in the proximal tubule reduces the ability of the proximal tubule to reabsorb bicarbonate. This retards the kidneys' ability to respond to acidosis by conserving bicarbonate and excreting an acid urine. When ECF volume is depleted, the resulting fall in GFR, rise in proximal tubular reabsorption, and increase in secretion of aldosterone combine to increase the conservation of bicarbonate and the excretion of acid. Thus, the kidneys' ability to respond to alkalosis by increasing the excretion of bicarbonate and reducing the excretion of acid is reduced.

These interrelationships are particularly important in the kidneys' response to loss of gastrointestinal secretions. In chronic vomiting, the continual loss of fluid containing H, Cl, and Na causes contraction of ECF volume and metabolic alkalosis. The response of the body to the volume contraction stimulates proximal tubular reabsorption, not only of salt and water but also of $NaHCO_3$. The reduced delivery of fluid to the distal segments of the nephron, coupled with the aldosterone stimulus of reabsorption, enhances bicarbonate reabsorption there also. This compromises the response to the alkalosis. If the ECF volume is returned to normal by administration of NaCl and water, the kidney can more easily correct the alkalosis.

The loss of intestinal secretions by diarrhea may produce metabolic acidosis. The accompanying loss of salt and water also causes ECF volume contraction. In this situation however, the response to the volume loss enhances the ability of the kidney to respond to the acidosis.

Another factor complicates the renal response to these acid-base disturbances. Potassium is lost in the vomitus and in the stool and hypokalemia may ensue. The consequent loss of potassium from cells, including tubular cells, stimulates H ion secretion (see Chapter 11). This also compromises the response to alkalosis and enhances the response to acidosis.

MEASUREMENT OF RENAL REACTION TO ACID-BASE IMBALANCES

An accurate assessment of the kidneys' contribution to maintaining acid-base balance necessitates the measurement of the results of Reactions 1, 2, and 3 in Figure 10-4. The rate of bicarbonate reabsorption, titratable acid formation, and ammonium excretion must be measured.

The amount of H ions that have combined with filtered HCO_3^- can be determined by the following equation:

$$T_{HCO_3} = P_{HCO_3} C_{in} - U_{HCO_3} \dot{V} \quad (\mu Eq/min)$$

To measure the amount of H ions combined with buffers such as phosphate, hydroxide is used to titrate the urine to blood pH. The titratable acid excretion rate, $U_{TA}\dot{V}$, can be calculated as follows:

$$U_{TA}\dot{V} = (\text{amount of } OH^- \text{ added/ml of urine})\dot{V} \quad (\mu Eq/min)$$

Since the pK of ammonium is so high, the addition of hydroxide to bring urine pH back to blood pH titrates little NH_4. Therefore, its concentration must be measured separately and the excretion rate calculated ($U_{NH_4} \dot{V}$ in $\mu Eq/min$).

The rate of total acid excretion is the result of both Reaction 2 and Reaction 3 in Figure 10-3.

$$\text{Acid excretion rate} = U_{TA}\dot{V} + U_{NH_4}\dot{V}$$

The mass of hydrogen ions secreted per min by the kidney = $T_{HCO_3} + U_{TA}\dot{V} + U_{NH_4}\dot{V}$

ALTERNATE CONCEPTS

Throughout this chapter we have emphasized the concept that the kidney contributes to the regulation of blood pH by excreting urine containing an excess of acid or alkali. It is our view that by removing that excess from the ECF the kidney returns blood pH to the control level.

Another conceptual approach emphasizes the kidney's addition of bicarbonate to blood. This approach considers that the kidney regulates the blood bicarbonate concentration. It states that the proximal tubule serves to reclaim filtered bicarbonate that would otherwise be lost and that the distal tubule and collecting tubule add "new" bicarbonate to blood by titrating phosphate and ammonia in tubular fluid.

We have chosen not to use this approach for the following reasons: First, the reaction of the kidney to respiratory acid-base disturbances drives the blood bicarbonate concentration away from the normal concentration as it restores blood pH to normal. Second, to state that the distal sections of the nephron add new bicarbonate to blood ignores the fact that bicarbonate is a labile ion and also ignores the presence of other major buffer systems in blood. Bicarbonate ions entering renal venous blood from tubular cells may be titrated to CO_2 by H ions (Reaction 1, Fig. 10-1). This alters the equilibrium of other buffer pairs such as Hb:HHb (Reaction 2, Fig. 10-1). The one common denominator to these reactions occurring in blood is the blood pH. We think it best to focus on how the kidneys react to maintain blood pH constant.

It is also common to determine quantitatively the kidneys' response to acid-base disturbances by measuring "net acid" excretion. Net acid excretion equals total acid excretion minus bicarbonate excretion. This is supposed to equal the *net* contribution of the kidney to restoration of acid-base balance. We do not believe this calculation to be correct. Consider the hypothetical situation in which the kidney happens to excrete a liter of glomerular filtrate with no change in its composition. It does not contain any titratable acid or alkali, since its pH is the same as blood, nor does it contain any ammonium. It does, however, contain 25 mEq of bicarbonate. Calculation of net acid excretion yields a value of -25 mEq. Yet the loss of that unchanged liter of glomerular filtrate would not change blood pH at all.

AMMONIUM

The ability of the kidney to produce and secrete the base NH_3 permits it to increase the buffer concentration of tubular fluid as the secretion of hydrogen ions reduces its pH. This enables the kidney to excrete additional acid in the form of NH_4.

Ammonia Production

The major precursor of ammonia is the amino acid glutamine, which contributes both its amide and amino nitrogen to the formation of ammonia. Ammonia is also produced from alanine and glycine.

Glutamine is extracted from both the blood and the tubular fluid by tubular cells. Within the mitochondria, glutamine is deamidated by the enzyme phosphate-dependent glutaminase (PDG) to glutamate and ammonia (Fig. 10-12). Glutamate can then be deaminated to α-ketoglutarate and ammonia by glutamate dehydrogenase (GDH) in the presence of nicotinamide adenine dinucleotide (NAD). Glycine and alanine may contribute their amino group to α-ketoglutarate by transamination to form glutamate, which can then be deaminated as indicated above.

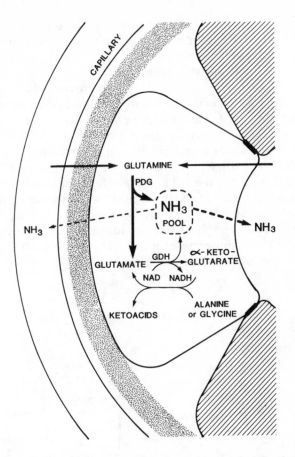

Figure 10-12.   The metabolic reactions involved in the renal production of ammonia. PDG = phosphate dependent glutaminase. GDH = glutamate dehydrogenase. NAD = nicotinamide adenine dinucleotide.

The interrelationships among these reactions are shown in Figure 10-12. The majority of the ammonium in the urine is obtained from deamidation of glutamine. The rest is obtained from deamination of glutamate and also from alanine and glycine.

Secretion of Ammonia

Ammonia exists in two forms. The base form, NH_3 (ammonia), is uncharged and lipid-soluble, so it easily and rapidly diffuses across cell membranes. The acid form, NH_4^+ (ammonium), is charged and lipid-insoluble, and cell membranes are impermeable to it. In solution, these two forms are in a dynamic equilibrium with H ions. As the H ion concentration increases (pH decreases), NH_3 is titrated to NH_4^+. The two forms of ammonium exist in equal concentration in a solution with a pH of 9, that is, the pK of ammonium is 9. The buffer equation, pH = pK + log $[NH_3]/[NH_4]$, indicates that the ratio of the two forms in a solution will decrease tenfold for each unit decrease in pH and that the ratio $[NH_3]/[NH_4]$ will equal 1/100 at a pH of 7.

The pH of tubular cells is thought to be approximately 7, and at that pH, only a small fraction of the total ammonium is in the permeant form, NH_3. Nevertheless, it is the concentration of NH_3 that is important because only NH_3 can easily diffuse out of the cell. Furthermore, because of the steady state that exists between H^+ and ammonia, NH_3 lost from the cell is immediately replaced by the dissociation of NH_4^+.

NH_3 can diffuse out of the cell into both the urine and the blood, and in those fluids it is titrated to NH_4^+. Figure 10-13A shows what happens as NH_3 diffuses into the tubular fluid. Nonionic NH_3 in the cell diffuses down a concentration gradient into the urine, where it combines with H to form the ionic, impermeant form, NH_4^+. In this latter form, it is "trapped" in the tubular fluid and cannot readily diffuse out. As NH_3

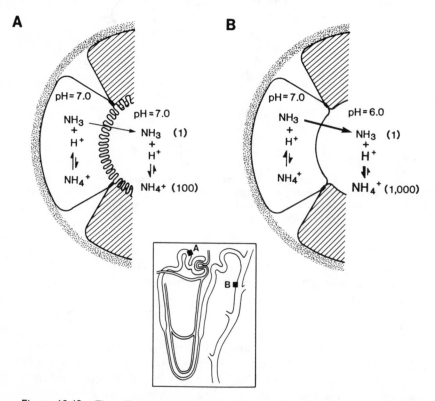

Figure 10-13. The effect of tubular fluid pH upon the secretion of NH_3 and the excretion of NH_4. The numbers indicate the relative concentrations of NH_3 and NH_4. (A) The addition of NH_3 to tubular fluid in the proximal tubule. (B) The addition of NH_3 to tubular fluid in the collecting tubule.

leaves the cell, NH_4^+ within the cell dissociates to replace it. Thus, a concentration gradient continually exists for NH_3 diffusion from the cell into the urine, until the concentration of NH_4 in the urine is sufficient to maintain the NH_3 concentration there at the level that exists in the cell. At that point, if the urine pH is 7, the ratio $[NH_3]/[NH_4]$ will equal 1/100.

Note that it is the concentration gradient for NH_3, not NH_4^+, that determines the rate of secretion. However, that concentration gradient is controlled by the pH of the tubular fluid. When H ion secretion by the tubular cells reduces the urine pH (Fig. 10-13B), the urine NH_3 concentration is reduced as it is titrated to NH_4^+. The concentration gradient between the cell and urine is then increased, and the rate of NH_3 diffusion into the urine rises. Much more NH_3 must enter the urine before the reaction with H ions allows the urine NH_3 concentration to equal that of the cell.

As Figure 10-13 indicates, if cell concentrations of NH_3 and H remain constant, the concentration of NH_4^+ in tubular urine should increase tenfold for each unit drop in pH (i.e., tenfold increase in ammonium concentration with a tenfold increase in H ion concentration). The theoretical rate of increase in NH_4^+ concentration as urine pH drops is indicated in Figure 10-14. In actuality, ammonium excretion does not increase that steeply when urine pH drops except in certain experimental situations. There are several reasons why the actual increase in concentration does not approach the theoretical. The major factor is the limited rate of ammonium production. At low urine pHs, the amount of NH_3 required to approach the theoretical limit is much more than the cells can produce.

Adaptation to Chronic Acidosis

It has been found that chronic acidosis of 2 to 3 days' duration increases the amount of ammonium excreted even when urine pH does not change (Fig. 10-14). This is due to a rise in the rate of ammonium production. Neither the stimulus nor the mechanism of this increase is known for certain. However it is caused, this stimulation of ammonium excretion increases the buffering capacity of the urine and allows the kidney to increase the excretion of acid.

Summary

Ammonium is produced in tubular cells mainly by the deamidation and deamination of glutamine. The lipid-soluble, uncharged form of ammonium, NH_3, diffuses into tubular fluid, where it combines with H ions to form charged, lipid-insoluble NH_4^+, which is trapped in the urine and excreted. When the urine pH is reduced by H ion secretion, NH_3 is titrated to NH_4^+, and this decrease in tubular fluid NH_3 concentration increases the diffusion of NH_3 from the cell into the urine.

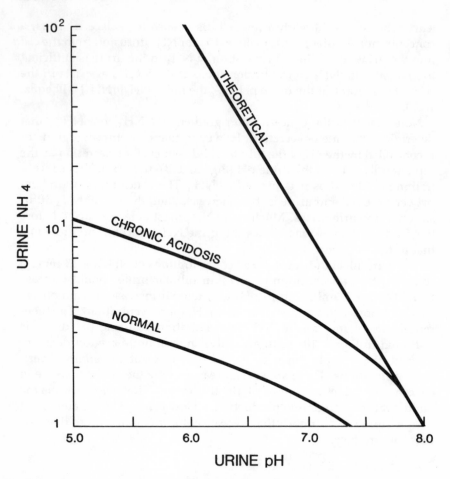

Figure 10-14. The effect of changes in urine pH on ammonium concentration in urine. Note that the ordinate is a log scale. The abscissa is linear, but it expresses hydrogen ion concentration in a log form.

The subsequent titration of NH_3 to NH_4^+ increases the total ammonium concentration in the urine. Chronic acidosis increases the rate of ammonium excretion, thereby permitting the kidney to excrete larger quantities of acid.

BIBLIOGRAPHY

General:

See the following chapters from: Brenner, B. M., and Rector, F. C., Jr., (Eds.): The Kidney. 2nd ed. Philadelphia, W. B. Saunders Co., 1981.
   Chapter 10. Warnock, D. G., and Rector, F. C., Jr.: Renal Acidification Mechanisms.
   Chapter 17. Cogan, M. G., Rector, F. C., Jr., and Seldin, D. W.: Acid-base Disorders.

Brenner, B. M., and Stein, J. H., (Eds.): Acid-Base and Potassium Homeostasis. Contemporary Issues in Nephrology. Vol. 2. New York, Churchill Livingstone, 1978.

Giebisch, G.: The Proximal Nephron. *In* Physiology of Membrane Disorders. Edited by T. E. Andreoli, J. F. Hoffman, and D. D. Fanestil, New York, Plenum Medical Book Co., 1978.

Specific:

Arruda, J. A. L., and Kurtzman, N. A.: Mechanisms and classification of deranged distal urinary acidification. Am. J. Physiol., *239* (Renal Fluid Electrolyte Physiol. *8*):F515, 1980.

Malnic, G.: CO_2 Equilibria in renal tissue. Am. J. Physiol., *239* (Renal Fluid and Electrolyte Physiol. *8*):F307, 1980.

Malnic, G., and Steinmetz, P. R.: Transport processes in urinary acidification. Kidney Internat., *9*:172, 1976.

Tannen, R. L.: Ammonia metabolism. Am. J. Physiol., *235* (Renal Fluid Electrolyte Physiol. *4*):F265, 1978.

CHAPTER 11

Maintenance of Potassium Balance

Maintenance of potassium balance is vitally important for normal nerve and muscle function. Both deficits and surfeits of potassium disturb the electrical activity of excitable membranes by altering the intracellular-to-extracellular potassium concentration ratio and by affecting membrane conductance to potassium. If loss of potassium is sufficient to cause significant hypokalemia, weakness of skeletal muscle ensues and eventually flaccid paralysis may occur. The effect on gastrointestinal smooth muscle can cause diarrhea and abdominal distension. Tachycardia and arrhythmias may develop in cardiac muscle. Deep tendon reflexes are diminished, and if the depletion is severe, a generalized areflexia can develop. Retention of excessive potassium may lead to hyperkalemia. The heart is particularly sensitive to hyperkalemia and progression to fatal cardiotoxicity can be unpredictable and often swift. Skeletal muscle weakness can also occur in hyperkalemia.

The body contains about 50 mEq of potassium per kg body weight. In a man weighing 70 kg this is approximately equivalent to 3500 mEq, 90% of which is contained in cells and is readily exchangeable. Only 2.5% is found in the extracellular fluid. Most of the rest is contained in bone. The normal range for the plasma potassium concentration is about 3.8 to 5.0 mEq/L. It is the most readily available clinical indicator of potassium balance, but it must be used with caution because it represents such a small fraction of the body content of potassium. Fractionally small losses or gains of potassium by cells can cause large changes in the plasma concentration. These shifts in and out of cells can easily occur in acid-base disorders, in disturbances of hormonal balance, and in response to a variety of drugs. The direction of the change in plasma concentration in these situations may not reflect the change in total body potassium.

Maintenance of an adequate intake of potassium is usually not a problem. Significant amounts occur in almost all foodstuffs and the normal diet contains 50 to 100 mEq per day. Only about 10% of the ingested potassium is normally lost in the stool. Thus, potassium balance is regulated primarily by controlling the rate of excretion by the kidneys, and this can be made to vary over a wide range. The normal rate of excretion, 50 to 100 mEq/day, is equivalent to about 5 to 15% of the filtration rate. However, the normal kidney can reduce the rate of excretion to as little as 5 mEq/day, and in some situations, can increase it to about 1000 mEq/day, which is equivalent to approximately 140% of the filtration rate. Thus, potassium is both reabsorbed and secreted by the tubular epithelium.

In normal circumstances, over 90% of the filtered load of K is reabsorbed by the proximal tubules and loops of Henle, and almost all K appearing in the urine has been secreted by the late distal tubules and collecting tubules. Thus, the rate of excretion is usually independent of the rate of filtration, but is closely tied to the rate of secretion. The major factor controlling the rate of secretion is apparently the concentration of K within the secreting cells.

This mechanism of excretion of the major *intracellular* cation can be contrasted to the mechanisms for excretion of the major *extracellular* cation. Na excretion is regulated by balancing the rates of filtration and reabsorption of large volumes of extracellular fluid. Changes in the rate of excretion occur in response to alterations in the composition and volume of the ECF. K excretion is relatively unaffected by filtration and reabsorption of extracellular fluid, but can be altered through the secretory process by changes in the composition of the intracellular fluid.

There are other interesting contrasts. The regulation of Na excretion is most efficient in conserving Na when intake is reduced, but is much less efficient in dealing with an excessive intake. However, the K excretory mechanisms can most effectively respond to an increased intake of K. Perhaps because of this, problems most often arise clinically from excessive retention of Na and excessive excretion of K. Despite these differences, the renal transport systems for Na and K are closely related in many ways.

TUBULAR SITES OF REABSORPTION AND SECRETION

Figure 11-1 shows the direction of K transport in the various segments of the nephron. Potassium and water are reabsorbed in the proximal tubule in the same proportion as they exist in the filtrate, that is, 60 to 70% of filtered K is reabsorbed and the concentration in the tubular fluid remains close to that of plasma.

Potassium is concentrated in the medullary ISF by a countercurrent process, but little is known about the mechanism of trapping. Potassium may be reabsorbed from the tubular fluid and added to the medullary ISF by the medullary sections of the collecting tubule. Countercurrent flow in the vasa recta may serve to trap it in the medulla and

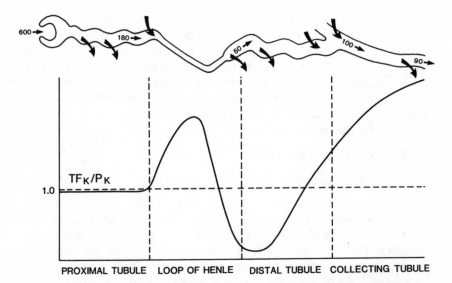

Figure 11-1. Tubular sites of potassium secretion and reabsorption. The numbers within the nephron indicate the average amount of potassium that reaches each segment of the nephron per day. The curve shows the changes in tubular fluid potassium concentration as both potassium and water are transported across the tubular epithelium.

increase its concentration in the ISF. From there it is thought that K diffuses into the descending limb of Henle's loop. Its concentration in fluid at the tip of the loop is much higher than in plasma (Fig. 11-1) and the amount reaching that site is greater than the amount filtered. However, K is extensively reabsorbed at some point along the ascending limb of Henle's loop, so that only 8 to 10% of the amount of K that was filtered reaches the distal tubule. The concentration in tubular fluid at that point is low.

The entire distal tubule evidently has the capacity to reabsorb K, and in states of K depletion, the concentration of K remains low along the full length of the distal tubule. Normally, however, K is secreted into the latter half of the distal tubule, where cells resembling those in the collecting tubule begin to appear (Chapter 5). The concentration of K and the amount in the tubular fluid in this segment can vary tremendously, depending on the physiologic status of the animal.

Potassium is also secreted by the cortical sections of the collecting tubule, causing the concentration and amount of K in tubular fluid to rise. However, it is usually reabsorbed to some extent in the medullary sections of the collecting duct. The rate of reabsorption is usually less than the rate of water reabsorption, so the concentration of K continues to rise. The possibility that this segment of the nephron also has the capacity to secrete K has not been eliminated.

The complexity of the pattern of K transport by the nephron, with the multiple sites of reabsorption and secretion, does not make experimentation or learning easy. It is helpful to recall, first, that about 90% of the filtered K is usually reabsorbed from the tubular fluid by the time it reaches the distal tubule; second, that variations in the rate of excretion are most often due to alterations in transport by tubular segments beyond that point; and, third, most of the changes in excretion are considered to be due to changes in the rate of secretion.

MECHANISMS OF TRANSPORT

Maintenance of Cellular Potassium Concentrations

All tubular cells, like most cells elsewhere in the body, maintain a high intracellular concentration of K. Moreover, the chemical gradient across the cell membrane is larger than the electrical gradient that opposes K diffusion out of the cell. This indicates that an active process utilizing metabolic energy transports K into the cell against the net electrochemical gradient (Fig. 1-6). The mechanism responsible for this is the Na-K-ATPase enzyme system (Fig. 1-8). Two findings indicate that the basolateral membrane is primarily responsible for maintaining a high cellular K concentration. First, the Na-K-ATPase enzyme system is located primarily in the basolateral membrane. Second, the cells maintain a normal K concentration when the tubular lumen is collapsed and transport across the apical membrane is abolished.

The cellular concentration of K is determined not only by the rate of active transport into the cell but also by the rate of movement out of the cell. Thus, another important factor governing the concentration of K in the cell is the permeability of the basolateral membrane to K.

Transepithelial Transport

Potassium transport across the basolateral membrane primarily determines its cellular concentration. However, the direction and rate of transepithelial transport of K are determined to a large extent by transport across the apical membrane. In the proximal tubule, K is probably actively transported into the cell across the apical membrane (Fig. 11-2). This reabsorptive process, like that for Na, is a gradient-limited mechanism. Passive diffusion of K in the opposite direction occurs not only across the apical membrane but also through the low-resistance paracellular pathway. In common with many of the other ionic transport systems in the proximal tubule, this is a high capacity, low gradient system. Because of the gradient limitation, its rate of reabsorption is highly dependent on the rate of water reabsorption.

Potassium movement into the lumen of the descending limb of Henle's loop or the pars recta of the proximal tubule is probably a passive process driven by a chemical gradient between the medullary ISF and the tubular fluid. The mechanism for K reabsorption in the

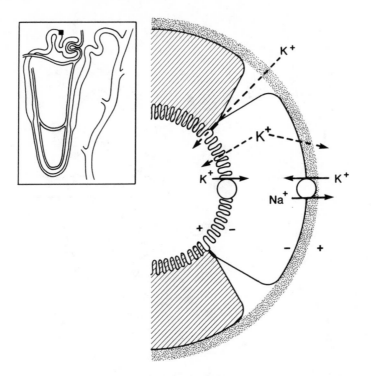

Figure 11-2. Potassium reabsorption in the proximal tubule.

ascending limb has not been directly studied. It does effectively remove K from the tubular fluid and reduces the concentration below the plasma concentration. The reabsorptive mechanism in the distal tubule can transport K against an electrochemical gradient. This process is probably initiated by active K transport across the apical membrane into the cell.

The mechanism of K secretion in the latter half of the distal tubule and in the collecting tubule has received the most attention from investigators, but there are still major gaps in our understanding of this process. It is clear that the process of secretion begins by active transport of K into the cell across the basolateral membrane (Fig. 11-3). The transport process that moves K from the cell across the apical membrane may be either active or passive. The electrical gradient opposing K diffusion from the cell into the lumen is small in that section of the nephron. Therefore, passive movement out of the cell down the *net* electrochemical gradient could account for much of the secretion of K. Yet, in the collecting tubule at least, that gradient is not always sufficient to account for the high concentrations found in the tubular fluid. This suggests the existence of an active mechanism in the apical membrane, transporting

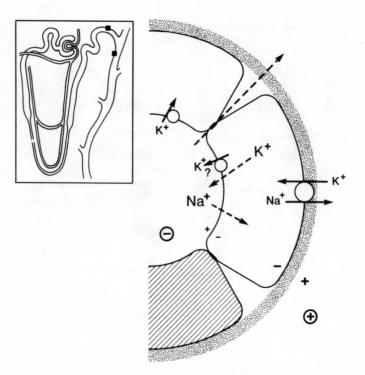

Figure 11-3. Mechanism of potassium secretion in the distal tubule and collecting tubule.

potassium into the lumen. Net secretion into the lumen may be limited either by an active or a passive reabsorptive flux. Thus secretion can be considered to be a gradient-limited transport process.

FACTORS AFFECTING EXCRETION

A variety of factors affect excretion of K, primarily by varying the rate of secretion. Some factors may alter K influx or efflux across the basolateral membrane, and in so doing, modify the cellular concentration so that the secretion rate rises or falls. Other factors may alter K fluxes across the apical membrane. For instance, the rate of secretion is sensitive to alterations in the composition of tubular fluid. Some of these changes probably modify the electrochemical gradient driving K movement across the apical membrane (Fig. 11-4).

Aldosterone

A rise in the plasma concentration of K stimulates secretion of aldosterone. It in turn stimulates secretion of potassium by the distal tubule and collecting tubule. The increase in secretion may be the result of a rise in uptake of K by the basolateral membrane, an increase in the potassium conductance of the apical membrane, or both.

Aldosterone secretion is increased by Na depletion, ECF volume contraction, and by other factors not related to K balance (see Chapter 9). In these instances, K losses may be excessive and K deficiency may result. Other factors, however, may limit the effect of aldosterone on K excretion in these situations (vide infra). There is no fixed relationship between the effects of aldosterone on Na reabsorption and K secretion. The effects of the hormone on the two processes can be separated by various means.

Spironolactone is a specific inhibitor of the the effect of aldosterone on tubular cells. Its use in situations in which aldosterone levels in blood are high reduces Na reabsorption and K secretion in the distal tubule and collecting tubule.

Dietary Factors

The rate of K secretion is sensitive to modifications in the dietary intake of K. The rate of secretion falls in response to dietary restriction

FACTORS THAT STIMULATE K$^+$ SECRETION

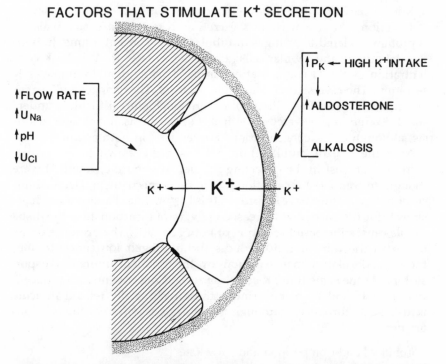

Figure 11-4. Factors that stimulate potassium secretion. On the right is a list of alterations in body fluid composition that stimulate secretion. On the left is a list of alterations in tubular fluid composition that modify the rate of secretion.

of K, but several days may be required to reduce the rate of excretion to the level of the rate of intake. The initial fall in excretion may be caused by a decrease in aldosterone secretion. However, the continued fall in excretion over a period of days is probably related to the decrease in the cellular concentration of K.

Increased intake of K is followed promptly by a rise in the rate of secretion. If the high intake is continued over a period of days, an adaptive response known as "potassium tolerance" occurs. This is characterized by an ability to survive acute potassium loads that would ordinarily be lethal. Apparently, both renal and extrarenal cells are able to take up K from the plasma more rapidly and the kidney is able to increase the rate of excretion more quickly and to a greater degree than is possible in normal circumstances. Adaptation to a high K diet is accompanied by an increase in renal Na-K-ATPase activity and an increase in cellular K concentrations. Part of these changes may be due to increased secretion of aldosterone.

Acid-Base Factors

Both respiratory and metabolic disturbances of acid-base balance lead to changes in K excretion that often are not appropriate for maintenance of K balance. Chronic metabolic alkalosis in particular can cause severe K depletion. The rise or fall in K excretion in *acute* acid-base imbalance is probably related to changes in tubular cell K concentrations. In both skeletal muscle and tubular cells, alkalosis increases the cellular K concentration as the H concentration drops. This evidently stimulates K secretion. The reverse occurs in acute acidosis. The changes in K excretion in *chronic* acid-base disturbances are much more difficult to understand. Excretion is elevated in both chronic alkalosis and chronic acidosis, although cell K concentrations are reduced in both circumstances.

An acute rise in tubular fluid pH has been shown to increase K secretion, at least in the collecting tubule. At one time, K and H were thought to compete for secretion by the same mechanism. Detailed micropuncture studies have disproven this hypothesis. These studies have shown, for instance, that increased delivery of bicarbonate to the distal tubule causes increased secretion of both H and K. The presence of the buffer in the tubular fluid reduces the hydrogen ion concentration, thereby stimulating net secretion by the gradient-limited transport system. At the same time, K secretion rises. Consequently, the concentration of H and K in the urine may be reciprocally related in acute acid-base disturbances, although the rates of secretion of the two ions are not.

Tubular Fluid Composition and Flow Rate

Changes in tubular fluid composition and flow rate have been shown to affect both secretion and reabsorption of potassium (Fig. 11-4). Inhibition of proximal tubular reabsorption of salt and water leads to reduced proximal reabsorption of K because of the gradient limitation. The rate of reabsorption in the thick ascending limb increases to some extent, but still an increased fraction of the filtered K escapes reabsorption. The rate of secretion is also augmented by the increased flow rate. This is partly explained by the following: A high flow rate continually sweeps secreted K away, preserving a low tubular fluid concentration. The low concentration maintains a high electrochemical gradient, favoring net secretion.

A high rate of secretion is also dependent on the maintenance of a favorable level of Na delivery to the K secretory sites. Normally, the concentration of Na in distal tubular fluid is high enough to maintain K secretion. However, the Na concentration in fluid reaching the collecting tubule frequently may be low enough to limit secretion. Diuresis caused by inhibition of salt and water reabsorption upstream may result in increased delivery of Na to the collecting tubule, thereby augmenting the rate of K secretion. This effect of Na may possibly be related to maintenance of normal pump activity in the basolateral membrane.

The chloride concentration in tubular fluid also affects K transport. A fall in the Cl concentration of the tubular fluid entering the distal sections of the nephron inhibits reabsorption and stimulates K secretion. This is particularly effective if the fall in Cl concentration is accompanied by normal or increased Na delivery to the sites of secretion. The mechanism for this Cl effect may be related to alteration of the electrical potential gradient across the apical membrane.

These changes in tubular fluid composition and flow rate can significantly affect the renal response to other factors affecting K excretion. The increase in K secretion in response to high blood levels of aldosterone depends greatly on an adequate tubular fluid flow rate and delivery of Na to the collecting tubule. The elevation of aldosterone levels in response to ECF volume contraction or Na depletion is often accompanied by a low rate of flow in the nephron and low Na concentration in the tubular fluid. This limits the effect of aldosterone on K excretion.

The loss of K that accompanies metabolic alkalosis may be limited if ECF volume depletion also occurs, since the tubular fluid Na concentration and flow rate are reduced in that circumstance. The loss of gastric secretions often causes hypochloremia as well as metabolic alkalosis. The subsequent reduction in tubular fluid Cl concentration may maintain a high rate of K excretion and prevent correction of the hypokalemia until chloride is administered.

Diuretics

Hypokalemia is a common, unwanted side effect accompanying chronic administration of diuretic agents. The effect of such agents on K secretion is apparent from the foregoing section. The increase in the Na concentration and flow rate of tubular fluid caused by these drugs stimulate K secretion in the distal tubule and collecting tubule. Furosemide has the additional effect of inhibiting K reabsorption in the thick ascending limb of Henle's loop. Carbonic anhydrase inhibitors such as acetazolamide also stimulate K secretion through their effect on cellular carbonic anhydrase. The resulting rise in cell pH stimulates K uptake across the basolateral membrane, causing further stimulation of secretion.

A few diuretic agents inhibit K secretion. Amiloride and triamterene, which cause only a modest diuresis by inhibiting Na reabsorption in the distal sections of the nephron, reduce K secretion. Spironolactone, as mentioned, will also decrease K secretion when aldosterone secretion is elevated.

BIBLIOGRAPHY

General:

See the following two chapters from: Brenner, B. M., and Rector, F. C., Jr., (Eds.): The Kidney. 2nd ed. Philadelphia, W. B. Saunders Co., 1981.
  Chapter 9. Giebisch, G., Malnic, G., and Berliner, R. W.: Renal Transport and Control of Potassium Excretion.
  Chapter 18. Cohen, J. J., Gennari, F. J., and Harrington, J. T.: Disorders of Potassium Balance.
Brenner, B. M., and Stein, J. H., (Eds.): Acid-Base and Potassium Homeostasis. Contemporary Issues in Nephrology. Vol. 2. New York, Churchill Livingstone, 1978.
Giebisch, G., and Stanton, B.: Potassium transport in the nephron. Ann. Rev. Physiol., 41:241, 1979.

Specific:

Bia, M. J., and DeFronzo, R. A.: Extrarenal potassium homeostasis. Am. J. Physiol., 240 (Renal Fluid Electrolyte Physiol. 9): F257, 1981.
Giebisch, G.: Some reflections on the mechanism of renal tubular potassium transport. Yale J. Biol. Med., 48:315, 1975.
Good, D. W., and Wright, F. S.: Luminal influences on potassium secretion: sodium concentration and fluid flow rate. Am. J. Physiol., 236 (Renal Fluid Electrolyte Physiol. 5): F192, 1979.
Grantham, J. J., Burg, M. B., and Orloff, J.: The Nature of transtubular Na and K transport in isolated renal collecting tubules. J. Clin. Invest., 49:1815, 1970.
Jamison, R. L., Sonnenberg, H., and Stein, J. H.: Questions and replies: role of the collecting tubule in fluid, sodium and potassium balance. Am. J. Physiol., 237 (Renal Fluid Electrolyte Physiol. 6): F247, 1979.
Sullivan, L. P., Welling, D. J., and Rome, L. A.: Effects of sodium and chloride on potassium transport by the bullfrog kidney. Am. J. Physiol., 240 (Renal Fluid Electrolyte Physiol. 9): F127, 1981.
Wright, F. S., and Giebisch, G.: Renal potassium transport: contributions of individual nephron segments and populations. Am. J. Physiol., 235 (Renal Fluid Electrolyte Physiol. 4): F515, 1978.

CHAPTER *12*

The Excretion of Calcium, Magnesium, and Phosphorus

CALCIUM

The kidneys are important in the regulation of the amount of calcium in the body and its concentration in the extracellular fluids. Calcium (Ca) has several important roles in the body. It is the principal crystalline mineral constituent of bone. Ionized Ca in the extracellular fluids is important in the process of blood coagulation, and in the control of neuromuscular excitability and muscular contraction. Intracellular Ca appears to have an important role in the mechanism of action of several hormones. The cytoplasmic levels of the cation are kept low (about $10^{-7}M$) by active Ca extrusion processes located in the plasma membranes.

Ca is ingested in the diet and absorbed principally in the small intestine. Adult humans normally absorb about 200 mg of Ca per day when given a diet containing approximately 1 g of Ca. Vitamin D increases the absorption of Ca from the intestines. During periods of rapid growth, as occur throughout childhood, a significant fraction of the absorbed Ca is deposited in bone. Thus, the urinary excretion of Ca is less than the amount absorbed through the intestines and the subject is in a state of "positive calcium balance." In adults, bone growth is curtailed and urinary Ca excretion "balances" the amount absorbed by the intestines.

The Ca level of the plasma determines to a major extent the release of parathyroid hormone (PTH) from the parathyroid glands. Decreased ionized Ca levels stimulate PTH release, whereas high Ca levels suppress the hormone. The normal plasma Ca concentration is 10 mg/dl, (5 mEq/L). Plasma proteins bind Ca, so that about 50 to 60% of the Ca in plasma is free and ultrafilterable. Approximately 10 g of Ca are filtered daily, of which 98% is reabsorbed by the renal tubules. Most of the Ca reabsorption occurs in the proximal tubules (about 60%), and the remainder in the ascending limb of Henle's loop and the distal nephron. Ca appears to be absorbed by active transport in all of these tubule segments.

The control of renal Ca excretion is not well understood. Most of the modulation of Ca excretion in normal persons is thought to occur by alterations in Ca reabsorption. Parathyroid hormone decreases, whereas corticosteroids increase renal Ca excretion.

The close correlation between urinary Na and Ca excretion in states associated with extracellular fluid volume expansion and contraction suggests that the renal transport of the two cations may be interconnected. This apparent coupling between Na and Ca absorption is most striking in the proximal tubule. However, in the distal tubule Na and Ca reabsorption may not be linked in the same way, since thiazide diuretics inhibit Na reabsorption and stimulate Ca reabsorption in this segment.

MAGNESIUM

Magnesium, like calcium, is present in bone, extracellular fluid, and inside cells. The levels of magnesium (Mg) in cells are much higher than those of Ca, possibly reflecting the fact that Mg is an essential cofactor for many intracellular enzymatic processes.

The plasma level of Mg is about 2.0 mEq/L, of which approximately 70 to 80% is ultrafilterable. Mg, again like Ca, is reabsorbed by the proximal renal tubules by a process that may be linked to the transport of Na. Altogether some 80 to 95% of the filtered Mg is reabsorbed by the renal tubules. The proximal tubules reabsorb about 20 to 30% of the filtered load, with 50 to 60% being absorbed in the loop of Henle. Parathyroid hormone increases Mg reabsorption in the loop of Henle. Recent evidence indicates that the loop of Henle may determine the rate of renal Mg excretion to a major extent.

PHOSPHORUS

Phosphorus (P) is found in the body in both organic and inorganic compounds. Although most of the phosphorus is in a crystalline state in the bones, the oxyanion derivative (phosphate) is an important factor in intracellular metabolism (adenosine triphosphate), hormone action (cyclic adenosine monophosphate), tissue oxygenation (2, 3 diphosphoglycerate), and renal acid excretion (phosphate buffers). Phosphorus is ingested in the diet, and eliminated in feces and urine. The kidneys play an important role in the day to day regulation of phosphorus balance.

The plasma phosphate level is about 2.5 to 4.5 mg/dl in normal adults (0.8 to 1.5 mM). Approximately 90% of the phosphate in plasma is unbound and thus free for filtration by the glomeruli. It subsequently undergoes extensive tubular reabsorption. Normally, less than 20% of the filtered load of phosphate is excreted in the urine. Most of the reabsorption occurs by active transport in the initial (S_1) portions of proximal tubules. The S_2 and S_3 segments of the proximal tubules and the cortical collecting tubules absorb only a small amount of phosphate. The absorption of phosphate in proximal tubules is not accompanied by significant leakage of the anion back into the tubular fluid; this is a capacity-limited rather than a gradient-limited transport system.

Phosphate is absorbed from the urine by a specific transporter located in the luminal plasma membrane. The movement of phosphate into the cytoplasm also depends on the presence of sodium ions in the tubule fluid, an example of a cotransport system driven by the sodium gradient. This gradient is ultimately dependent on the Na-K-ATPase in the basolateral membrane (the sodium pump).

Parathyroid hormone increases renal phosphate excretion by inhibiting reabsorption of the anion in the proximal tubules. Conversely, the activated forms of vitamin D (25-hydroxycholecalciferol and 1, 25-dihydrocholecalciferol) increase the renal reabsorption of phosphate.

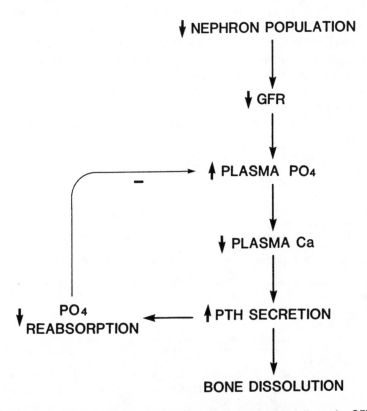

Figure 12-1. The "trade-off hypothesis" in chronic renal failure. As GFR falls steadily, factors are set into play to maintain phosphate balance.

Urinary excretion changes promptly in relation to the dietary load of phosphate. A "high" phosphate diet decreases the reabsorption of this anion by the proximal tubules, whereas phosphate-restricted diets cause nearly complete reabsorption of filtered phosphate. These adaptive changes do not appear to depend on modifications in circulating levels of parathyroid hormone or vitamin D.

The consequences of ineffective regulation of phosphate excretion are dramatic in individuals with progressive renal insufficiency. The fall in phosphate excretion leads to high levels of parathyroid hormone (PTH), which causes bone dissolution. This occurs in the following way (Fig. 12-1): The fall in functioning nephron population reduces GFR, which decreases the rate of phosphate excretion and raises the plasma PO_4 concentration. This causes deposition of calcium phosphate salts in tissues and the plasma Ca concentration falls. PTH secretion is stimulated by the decrease in blood Ca levels, and the increased PTH tends to reduce PO_4 reabsorption, so that the rise in plasma PO_4 concentration is countered to some extent. However, the increased levels of PTH also stimulate bone dissolution. This cyclic process is replayed continuously as the GFR falls steadily due to the chronic disease process and ultimately leads to high circulating levels of parathyroid hormone. Thus, the patient is able to maintain normal phosphate balance as GFR falls, but in the long run, the increasing levels of PTH are deleterious, since this hormone promotes the dissolution of bone calcium salts. This process is referred to as the "trade-off hypothesis," whereby plasma levels of ionic phosphate and Ca are maintained reasonably normal during the evolution of renal insufficiency at the expense of progressive bone destruction.

BIBLIOGRAPHY

General:

Dennis, V. W., Stead, W. W., and Myers, J. L.: Renal handling of phosphate and calcium. Ann. Rev. Physiol., 41:257, 1979.

Quamme, G. A., and Dirks, J. H.: Magnesium transport in the nephron. Am. J. Physiol., 239 (Renal Fluid Electrolyte Physiol. 8): F393, 1980.

Suki, W.: Calcium transport in the nephron. Am. J. Physiol., 237 (Renal Fluid Electrolyte Physiol. 6): F1, 1979.

Ullrich, K. J.: Sugar, amino acid, and Na^+ co-transport in the proximal tubule. Ann. Rev. Physiol., 41:181, 1979.

Specific:

Dennis, V. W., and Brazy, P. C.: Sodium, phosphate, glucose, bicarbonate and alanine interactions in the isolated proximal convoluted tubule of the rabbit kidney. J. Clin. Invest., 62:387, 1978.

Dennis, V. W., Woodhall, P. B., and Robinson, R. R.: Characteristics of phosphate transport in isolated proximal tubule. Am. J. Physiol., 231:979, 1976.

CHAPTER 13

Diuretics

The kidneys normally regulate the excretion of NaCl and water so precisely that the body content of water, and its partitioning between intracellular and interstitial compartments, is maintained in a steady state. In some clinical conditions (e.g., congestive heart failure and liver disease) the kidneys do not excrete a quantity of NaCl equal to that ingested. This retention of salt obligates the retention of water, and the NaCl and water content of the body increases. Since NaCl is the major osmotically active solute in the interstitial fluid, the volume of this compartment increases primarily.

The "error" in renal salt excretion does not have to be very large over a relatively long period of time to cause severe fluid retention and edema. Normal man filters about 150 to 180 L of extracellular fluid per day, of which all but about 1%, or 1.5 L, is reabsorbed by the renal tubules (Chapter 7). If the kidneys make only a 0.5% "error" in reabsorption, i.e., 99.5% of the filtered salt and water is reabsorbed in the face of a constant fluid intake, then the subject will retain about 0.75 L of water each day. In one week, 5.25 L of extra water will be retained, which is a weight gain of about 11.5 pounds. Thus, small "errors" in the reabsorption of salt and water can build up to large excesses of body water. This fluid tends to accumulate as edema in the dependent parts of the body and in body cavities, such as the peritoneal and thoracic spaces.

To overcome the abnormal accumulation of salt and water in patients, several chemical substances have been developed that decrease tubular NaCl reabsorption in different parts of the nephron. Since these substances increase the rate of urine flow (diuresis), they are known collectively as diuretics. Most diuretics act *primarily* to decrease the reabsorption of Na or Cl (saliuresis, natriuresis, chloruresis); the increased water excretion is *secondary* to the increased excretion of salt. The unreabsorbed salts in the urine cause the increased excretion of water by mechanisms described in Chapters 7 and 8.

EFFECT OF DIURETICS ON THE INDIVIDUAL SEGMENTS OF THE NEPHRON.

Proximal tubule

Solutes and water are reabsorbed in isotonic proportions in the proximal tubule. A significant fraction of Na reabsorption is dependent on the reabsorption of bicarbonate from the tubule fluid (Chapter 7). Acetazolamide and derivatives of this drug inhibit carbonic anhydrase, an enzyme in the proximal tubule that plays a key role in renal H secretion and HCO_3 reabsorption (Chapter 10). Inhibition of the enzyme leads to a decrease in bicarbonate reabsorption, and secondarily, Na is constrained within the tubule fluid to maintain electroneutrality. Acetazolamide, therefore, increases the amount of bicarbonate-rich tubular fluid leaving the proximal tubule. Normally, $NaHCO_3$ is poorly reabsorbed by the more distal parts of the nephron (especially so when acetazolamide inhibits the small amount of carbonic anhydrase in distal segments), and the loss of $NaHCO_3$ obligates the excretion of other solutes and water in the urine.

By causing $NaHCO_3$ loss, acetazolamide can, with time, cause systemic acidosis and, therefore, is not useful clinically for long term management of patients who have a primary defect in the excretion of NaCl. Several other drugs can inhibit NaCl reabsorption in the proximal tubule (furosemide, mercurials, thiazides), but only when present in the blood in concentrations that are too high to be clinically useful.

Loop of Henle

Sodium chloride is reabsorbed without water in the ascending limb of Henle's Loop. Furosemide and ethacrynic acid act specifically on this segment to decrease NaCl reabsorption and are most effective when applied to the luminal surface of the cells (Fig. 13-1). Both of these drugs are significantly bound to plasma proteins and are poorly filtered. However, a unique system delivers effective concentrations of these two drugs to their site of action (Fig. 13-1). The organic anion transport mechanism in the proximal tubule secretes the drugs into the tubular fluid, and they are carried to the ascending limb in that fluid stream. Since this delivery system can raise the concentration of the drugs in tubular fluid several-fold higher than in plasma, small doses of the drugs can be used and plasma concentrations can be maintained at levels that do not affect other organs.

The mechanism of inhibition by furosemide and ethacrynic acid probably involves the specific blockade of a sodium-chloride symport mechanism in the urinary membrane of the ascending limb cells (Fig. 13-1). Cl transport is decreased primarily since Na can enter the cell by other means, but Na is constrained in the tubular fluid to preserve electroneutrality, leading to an increased delivery of salt out of the ascending limb.

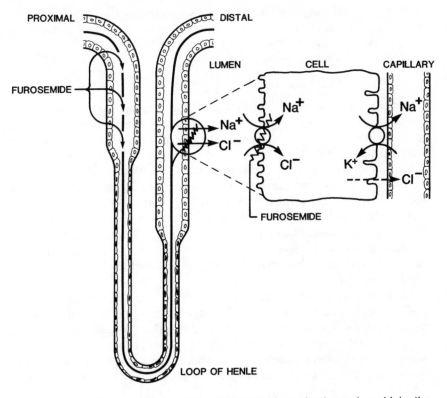

Figure 13-1. Mechanism of action of furosemide and ethacrynic acid in the nephron.

Certain organic molecules containing mercury (meralluride and mersalyl) also interfere with salt reabsorption in the ascending limb by a mechanism similar to that for furosemide and ethacrynic acid. These so-called mercurial diuretics were among the first potent diuretics to be used clinically, but they can be toxic and must be administered parenterally. They have been supplanted by the newer agents that are safer and effective when administered orally.

Distal Tubule

Sodium chloride is absorbed in the distal tubule with varying amounts of water. This reabsorption can be blocked by thiazide diuretics, which are derivatives of the sulfonamide group of drugs ($R-SO_2-NH_2$) that have less carbonic anhydrase-inhibiting capacity than the parent compounds, sulfanilamide and acetazolamide. The mechanism of action of the thiazides (chlorothiazide, hydrochlorothiazide, chlorthalidone, and metolazone) is not completely understood.

Two other compounds not belonging to the thiazide group, amiloride and triamterene, also inhibit salt reabsorption in the cortical distal segments by interfering with *sodium* transport across the luminal membrane. This is in contrast to the action of furosemide and ethacrynic acid, which primarily block the transport of *chloride* in the luminal membrane of the ascending limb.

Collecting Tubules and Ducts

Sodium chloride is reabsorbed with varying amounts of water in collecting tubules and ducts. The magnitude of salt reabsorption is strongly dependent on the plasma level of aldosterone, which also stimulates K secretion (Chapter 9). Spironolactone is a competitive inhibitor of aldosterone. By interfering with the effect of aldosterone on tubular cells, this drug diminishes the rate of NaCl reabsorption and K secretion in the distal tubule and collecting segments.

Triamterene and amiloride also retard NaCl reabsorption and K secretion in these segments by directly diminishing Na transport across the luminal membrane. Spironolactone, triamterene, and amiloride are rather "weak" diuretics usually used in conjunction with drugs that have a more proximal site of action.

Since furosemide and ethacrynic acid decrease salt transport in the medullary structures, these diuretics alter the composition of the medullary interstitial fluid and the tubular fluid entering the collecting system. This diminishes the osmotic gradient for water reabsorption from late segments of the distal tubules, the collecting tubules, and ducts, and net water absorption is reduced despite the presence of adequate levels of ADH.

GENERAL PRINCIPLES OF DIURETIC ACTION

It is important to realize that tubular segments distal to the site of action of a diuretic agent are able to compensate to a limited extent for the inhibition of salt and water reabsorption upstream. For instance, the inhibition of salt reabsorption in the loop of Henle by furosemide is partially compensated by increased reabsorption of salt in the distal and collecting tubules. The means by which this compensation occurs is illustrated in Figure 7-11. This compensation of the potent effect of furosemide is limited and a large fraction of the salt that escapes reabsorption in the loop of Henle appears in the final urine. Weaker diuretics may partially inhibit local reabsorption only to have a large fraction of unreabsorbed NaCl recaptured further downstream.

It is even more important to appreciate the segmental action of diuretics during chronic usage. When furosemide is given to a patient, there is a rapid increase in urine flow rate and a decrease in body weight. (Body weight changes provide a reasonable indication of changes in body water content over relatively short intervals of observation.) When the drug is given for several days in succession, there is a gradual return in the rate of urine flow and NaCl excretion to the values

TABLE I   PRINCIPAL TUBULAR SITES OF DIURETIC ACTION

Tubular Segment	Drug
Proximal tubule	Acetazolamide
Ascending limb of Henle	Furosemide Ethacrynic acid Mercurials
Distal Tubule	Chlorothiazide Metolazone Triamterene Amiloride
Collecting System	Amiloride Triamterene Spironolactone

seen before the diuretic was begun (Fig. 13-2). This is reflected by a stabilization of body weight. In other words, the subject is brought into a state of water balance, but at a lower absolute content of body water. It may appear that the drug is no longer working properly because the diuresis has been curtailed. However, the diuretic is certainly working in this example, because the body weight (body water) is being maintained at a reduced value. What has happened is that a complex series of intrarenal adjustments have been activated to prevent the relentless loss of body salt and water due to the diuretic. This is referred to as the "braking phenomenon," and is a reflection of the fact that some segments of the renal tubule (primarily proximal tubule) are reabsorbing NaCl at an increased rate equal to the degree of inhibition (caused by furosemide) in the ascending limb. Were it not for the "braking phenomenon," subjects would lose body salt and water to the point of severe dehydration, in which case GFR would fall to a low level.

The mechanism of the "braking phenomenon" is illustrated in Figure 13-2. As body water (specifically plasma volume) decreases, the proximal tubules, which are not inhibited by the low plasma levels of furosemide, reabsorb increased amounts of salt and water. Gradually, the delivery of salt and water to the ascending limb is reduced. Consequently, the inhibition of reabsorption of a much smaller amount of salt presented to the ascending limb leads to a reduction in the excretion of salt in the urine so that it is once more equal to that ingested in the diet. In this way, salt and water balance is reestablished. Although not shown in Figure 13-2, some compensatory increases in salt and water reabsorption probably also occur in the distal tubule and the collecting

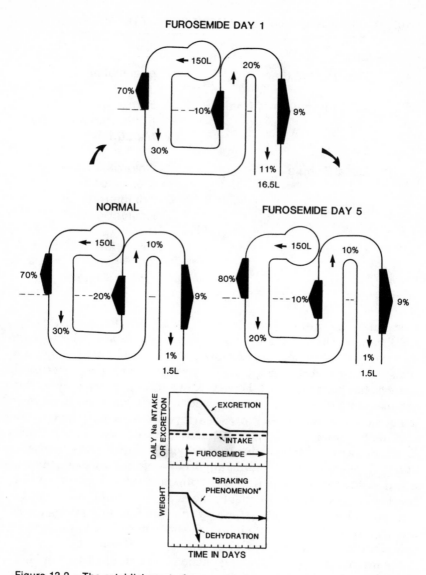

Figure 13-2. The establishment of a new steady-state for fluid balance during the administration of furosemide. Water excretion is shown in liters, and sodium reabsorption and excretion in percent of the filtered load. This diagram emphasizes the changes that occur in salt reabsorption in the proximal tubule to account for the attainment of salt and water balance.

system as a part of the "braking phenomenon." The "braking phenomenon" is probably activated for all diuretics that do not block salt and water reabsorption in the proximal tubule.

As one can see, the relative "strength" of a diuretic is reflected to some degree by the rate of urine flow only when the drug is given acutely. Over short intervals one can expect that for each 1% decrease in net tubule NaCl reabsorption about 1.5 L of extra urine will be excreted per day. Thus, a diuretic need only inhibit salt reabsorption by a few percent to cause an impressive increase in urine flow rate.

EFFECTS ON POTASSIUM EXCRETION

Several diuretics inhibit potassium reabsorption in specific tubule segments (acetazolamide in proximal tubules, furosemide and ethacrynic acid in the ascending limb) and indirectly stimulate secretion in the late distal tubule and collecting tubules. Others inhibit potassium secretion in the distal nephron (amiloride, triamterene, spironolactone).

Diuretics that act proximal to the collecting system cause increased amounts of NaCl and water to flow past the distal K secretory sites (Chapter 11). This increases the secretion of K, and in some instances, can lead to severe K deficiency.

OTHER EFFECTS

Thiazide diuretics decrease the renal excretion of calcium, whereas furosemide is calciuric.Thiazides, amiloride, triamterene, and spironolactone do not directly interfere with urinary concentrating capacity, whereas furosemide and ethacrynic acid impair the concentration process.

With chronic usage, the fractional excretion of urate is decreased and the plasma level of this organic anion is usually increased in patients receiving diuretics in effective doses. The diminished renal excretion rate is probably due to increased reabsorption of urate in the proximal tubules, a further reflection of the "braking phenomenon." In other words, the increased reabsorption of salt and water in the proximal tubule caused by chronic extracellular fluid volume contraction is accompanied by an increased rate of urate reabsorption in these segments (see Chapter 6).

Demeclocycline and lithium cause a water diuresis by inhibiting the action of vasopressin in the collecting system. These drugs apparently have no effect on renal salt excretion.

BIBLIOGRAPHY

General:

Grantham, J. J., and Chonko, A. M.: The Physiological Basis and Clinical Use of Diuretics. *In* Sodium and Water Homeostasis. Edited by B. M. Brenner, and J. H. Stein, Contemporary Issues in Nephrology. Vol. 1. New York, Churchill Livingstone, 1978.

Mudge, G. H.: Diuretics and Other Agents Employed in the Mobilization of Edema. *In* The Pharmacological Basis of Therapeutics. 6th ed. Edited by A. G. Gilman, L. S. Goodman, and A. Gilman. New York, Macmillan Publishing Co. Inc., 1980.

Reineck, H. J., and Stein, J. H.: Mechanisms of Action and Clinical Uses of Diuretics. *In* The Kidney. 2nd ed. Edited by B. M. Brenner, and F. C. Rector, Jr. Philadelphia, W. B. Saunders Co., 1981.

Specific:

Burg, M. B., Stoner, L., Cardinal, J., and Green, N.: Furosemide effect on isolated perfused tubules. Am. J. Physiol., *225:*119, 1973.

Edelman, I. S., Bogoroch, R., and Porter, G. A.: On the mechanism of action of aldosterone on sodium transport. The role of protein synthesis. Proc. Natl. Acad. Sci. U.S.A., *50:*1169, 1963.

Liddle, G.: Aldosterone antagonists and triamterene. Ann. N.Y. Acad. Sci., *139:*466, 1966.

Rocha, A. S., and Kokko, J. P.: Sodium, chloride and water transport in the medullary thick ascending limb of Henle: Evidence for active chloride transport. J. Clin. Invest., *52:*612, 1973.

Suki, W., Rector, F. C. Jr., and Seldin, D. W.: The site of action of furosemide and other sulfonamide diuretics in the dog. J. Clin. Invest., *44:*1458, 1965.

"What is man, when you come to think upon him, but a minutely set, ingenious machine for turning, with infinite artfulness, the red wine of Shiraz into urine?"

Isak Dinesen

INDEX

Page numbers in *italics* indicate illustrations; numbers followed by "t" refer to tables.